A POET'S SURVIVAL JOURNAL IN THE COVID-19 PANDEMIC

A POET'S SURVIVAL JOURNAL IN THE COVID-19 PANDEMIC

Mind, Body and Soul Reflections

ROSALINDA RUIZ SCARFUTO

Re-Bound Publishing

Contents

ISBN 978-0-578-74228-1 ISBN Perfect bound
ISBN 978-0-578-74226-7 E-book

First Edition, August 2020

To Mother Earth
Humanity
Birds, Bees & Butterflies

Acknowledgements

I would to thank family, friends, mentors and gardeners; especially María Jesús, Eloísa, Pak Ketut, Ibu Ketut, Putu, Denise, Bob, Elena, Tony, Kristin, Luca, Jean E., Mary Ellen, Margo, Richard, James, Jan, Bruce, Penny, Diane, Marina, Harold, Madeline, José Luis, Yolanda, Marta, Pepe, Doug, Inés, Cayetano, Abraham, Betsy, Emma, Ramon, Angela, Bruno, Gustavo, Julie, Jesús, Andrea, Michelle, Gloria, Gabriella, Joyce, Charlotte, Joanie, Marie, Karen, Susana, Cristina, Luisa, María, Josué, Robert, Henning, Isabel, Maceline, Samuel, Javier, Clemencia, Pilar, Charo, Ana, Abby, Mimi, George, Paul, Carmen, Michael, Carlos, Félix, Candy, Eduardo, Juan Pablo, Alejandro, Paco, José, Antonio, Manolo, Flora, Silvia and Nesto.

Introducción (español)

En su conjunto, el libro ofrece en igual medida consuelo y una guía de supervivencia. Se divide en dos formatos diferentes para un público más amplio, uno en poesía y otro en prosa, que cuentan la misma historia en paralelo. La sección de poesía no ha sido traducida ya que habría sido muy difícil transmitir la verdadera esencia y humor dada la limitación de tiempo para esta primera edición. En el futuro, puede que sea posible. En resumen, una traducción de la sección de poesía habría restado tiempo y energía de su publicación a tiempo. Por lo tanto, la encontrarán solo en su formato original.

Sin embargo, la poesía va acompañada y contextualizada a través de la sección equivalente del libro llamada 'Mi aprendizaje', que se presenta aquí en español. Rosalinda consideró que esta sección era de vital importancia que estuviese disponible sin demora alguna como valor añadido para los hispanohablantes. Esta sección trata principalmente de la reacción de su cuerpo al Covid-19 así como de consejos sobre cómo lo afrontó ella durante seis semanas. Además, explica la mentalidad que le permitió mantenerse centrada y básicamente permanecer tranquila durante todo el período del virus, mientras estaba en casa aislada. Es una historia personal que abarca desde la aparición del virus, pasando por el punto álgido del ataque del virus y finalmente el desafiante camino a la recuperación.

Rosalinda Ruiz Scarfuto, PhD is a native Californian, published poet, multimedia artist. She is a poet-painter and researcher investigating the 3D poetic canvas with tactile perception. Rosalinda began her artistic career with ceramics and poetry. She has lived and traveled from Japan to Spain walking the land including the Himalayas and Kenyan bush. Her first trip around the world was a 5-year sojourn completed by the age of 26. Over the years she has continued studying ceramics adding photography, Hanga, painting and jazz to her repertoire. Her prolonged stays in Asia fostered her Buddhist philosophy. Rosalinda is never far from her roots in California and is available for international workshops about the Forest Flaneur methodology she developed in her doctoral thesis including creative writing, painting, and mindfulness. She enjoys her organic garden and yoga in her free time.

I

Forward

Poetry and practicality merge in this individual journey through the Covid19 pandemic 2020. After successfully completing a practice-based PhD published as '*The Forest Flaneur*', Rosalinda was living and working in Madrid when the Coronavirus hit Europe shaking 21st Century life by the scruff of its neck. The ongoing hustle of self-employment, overcrowded public transport, rushed meal breaks – all the familiar stresses and strains of metropolitan life. Then it all stopped. Lockdown hit, the virus was HERE, and Rosalinda contracted it. Facing the virus through art, poetry, yoga, humour and love, Rosalinda wrote her way back to her characteristic, vigorous and healthy self.

As a whole the book offers solace and survival guide in equal measure. The poetic chapters, written intensively while going through the peak of the virus attack, have a surreal quality approaching automatic writing. The poetry is companioned and contextualized through the parallel 'What I learned' sections of the book.

These sections deal with everything from sleep and toilet moments to body, soul and heart nourishment. Advice and encouragement are freely given on how to nurse and nurture self through the challenges and changes of Covid19 independently of a medical support system, which is, in fact, how most people on the planet will have to get through it.

This account of personal experience stands incontrovertibly against an international confusion of science/pseudo-science, conspiracy theory, death and economic havoc.

Rosalinda's positive, humorous and quirky approach to surviving and thriving in the pandemic is invaluable and accessible to every reader. It will stand unarguably as a historically important text written at an extraordinary time in human existence.

Dr Angela Thwaites, London, July 2020
Artist-Researcher

II

Preface

COVID-19, previously known as the 2019 novel coronavirus, struck the world in 2020 and has changed the lives of millions of people. Now, those of you that have not been infected and do not have a family member or a close friend that overcame the virus: Have you ever wondered what survivors of this deadly virus have had to overcome? Those who have recovered from the virus: Can you explain with great detail your experience in battling this extremely contagious virus?

Rosalinda not only describes with poetry and prose the five weeks of her personal battle with the virus, but gives us a guideline of her recovery. This ingenious author transformed her struggles and pain into poetry in order to vanquish the novel coronavirus. Rosalinda integrated art and science in this magnificent book that will definitely help you understand and describe all of the symptoms, tribulations, pains, and emotional stress a person with COVID-19 must defeat.

Rosalinda's poetry takes the reader through real feelings, like we say in Spanish: "En carne propia" (in one's own flesh). COVID-19 becomes more precise and will be fully understood with the detailed descriptions of every symptom she provides through her beautifully written prose. Rosalinda also profoundly researched how this virus attacks the different body parts and affects their functions. Her personal account will also teach the reader how to counter-attack this powerful virus in natural ways, using the body, mind, and soul.

This brave author had the courage to overcome, learn, and now teach us how to battle this virus head on, without the use of any medications. She even describes a lot of her natural teas and scientifically backs up every herb, vegetable, and fruit she used to boost her immune system. I am definitely adding some of the teas she used for her recovery. For example, I am going to buy turmeric, something I have never used. Also, I will start using the horsetail that grows in my backyard.

This book has transformed the way I thought about COVID-19. One of the greatest lessons I learned from Rosalinda's journey is the importance to integrate and empower one's mind, body and soul to overcome any illness or obstacle that comes across your life. I now know how scary and powerful this virus is, so I am going to get my body, mind and soul stronger in case this or any other virus enters my life.

Ramón Silva Ruelas, California-USA, July 2020
Tonatiuh- "Danzantes del Quinto Sol" (Founder)

1

Author's Introduction

I have to admit I have never been in an emergency other than earthquakes. When the San Francisco Bay Bridge collapsed, I was standing under the threshold of my house nearby, watching the Earth move. It was a wave on the horizon and quite a strange sense for a matter of seconds. Days after the event we were paralyzed with no electricity and normal life was temporarily put on hold. However, this virus marked me like a tattoo, forever.

Hindsight 2020
Navigating unchartered waters!

On an early Spring day in March, I found myself in the middle of a pandemic and unknowingly at an epicenter in Madrid, Spain. I realize now that many of those who are untouched by the Covid-19 personally seem to feel it is a mystery out there somewhere. I suppose I would have the same impression if circumstances had played out differently.

In fact, right up until March 8th, I remember thinking that Italy was overreacting by cancelling the Women's March as relayed to me by a long-time friend living near Milan. Three days later, March 11th, Madrid was starting its lockdown. I recall riding the commuter train and everyone was chatting about the government sudden announcement of school closure to begin in 24 hours. Stepping off the train and into the station, I noticed people were moving with purpose. It occurred to me that it was pertinent to get home and grab the shopping cart and head to the store.

It overcame us like a heat wave in a small dusty town in the South of Spain, heavy and unbearably forceful pressure mounting with each hour. At this point I was feeling perfectly fine. The grocery store was full of people with large quantities of food, supplies, and toilet paper. I had my small cart and could only carry what fit into it with a bag on my shoulder as reserve. It was sunny and nice afternoon, so I took advantage of the weather to go for a bike ride. Days in Spring can vary and we were coming out of a cold spell, so the warm breeze was a welcome to distract me.

2

Self Quarantine Hits Me

Self-quarantine hits me like a slap in the face.
How did I get from cruising on my bicycle to collapse in 24 hours?

I am extremely grateful for constant contact with family, friends, and my medical advisors (western and eastern) to have been able to sustain a homebound recovery avoiding hospitalization. Self-quarantine means isolation and complete care by yourself. I have to admit years of yoga training and discipline given at a young age helped tremendously to keep my brain on target, even when it was failing to respond from lack of oxygen or swelling. Tidbits of news from Wuhan also helped to put the virus into perspective, especially one report of a British overseas resident who reported that he had had a cold one day and then suddenly he came down with pneumonia and was rushed to the hospital with respiratory complications. I finally admitted to my fever after that lovely bike ride around the river and the mega shopping spree. I now think back on how lucky I was in preparing my house with supplies that would have to last me three weeks. Actually, I had only thought about

10 days-worth of fresh fruits and vegetables to hold out for the original lockdown scheduled by the government. Nevertheless, I stocked up on beans, rice and sardines just in case for more days reminiscing about other emergencies. No sooner had I realized I had a fever on Friday 13th was I bedridden with excruciating pain in my kidneys and legs. Dehydration set in rapidly and I became so weak I could not even plan a meal, so I just forwent the effort. I was advised by friends to avoid aspirin and try to fight it off with my own immune system. This was in line with my own philosophy about illness, so I obliged. Reports were varied on the outcome of aspirin related drugs, so I suffered the next 5 days with the virus alone in my apartment. At this point, it was inevitable, I had to self-quarantine for 14 days, even after the fever subsided. In turn, I began to ration my food and toilet paper.

3

Cocoon to Butterfly

I invite you to my journey of metamorphosis.

I began this journey on a train commuting from Madrid, a major European capital and an epicenter of Covid 19 to a rural town nearby. After living in several urban capitals around the world, full of vibrant challenges and new experiences (Tokyo, Bangkok, San Francisco, etc.), a small virus opened my eyes wider and quicker than any other situation I had come up against in life. It was a novel bullet train with its own fast forward time frame, and I hung on to the handrail gasping for air as it passed through a dark tunnel. I felt as though I was headed to an abyss, like a never-ending story. My body was its playground and I had no control over where it would attack. I just had to ride the wave, a heat wave, dry and dusty. I began to write this poetry book for two reasons: 1) recovery therapy to put my thoughts on paper to capture the experience and 2) to offer encouragement to others to confront the virus at home without hospitalization.

The transition from an urban dweller to a part-time organic farmer was the result of this journey. I literally have no desire to step foot in an urban center and quite frankly it scares me as I associate the city life with health risks. I am sure this is a reaction to a harsh reality and may change in the future. However, I found I craved sunshine and fresh air after the ordeal that lasted approximately 6 weeks. My muscle mass dropped tremendously and I lost almost 9 kilos (20 pounds) in 3 weeks. I had to relearn how to walk and regain strength in all my organs. Then I had to relearn how to eat in order to keep my "ideal" weight. It was one of the positive side effects. I rented a plot of land to start a garden after finding plants to be a source of comfort in my apartment on the sunny back terrace during quarantine. Silence was the best way to recover and noise levels were highly reduced during lockdown. I am sure with ayurvedic teas during the virus and yoga pranayama for recovery combined with being in touch with nature can highly affect anyone faced with this type of virus or other life threat.

My butterfly wings emerged from a state of crystallization, so grateful.

4

Naïve Commuter

I had just bought my bicycle to venture into the countryside in my free time. I felt a slight fever or not? I peddled home. I thought, it was just the change in the weather. It was an early spring, warm day that was signaling a new season. Who would know that my bike ride was more precious than expected? My last memory of being outside, carefree and welcoming Spring 2020.

Innocence is Bliss?

It seems as though,
though never seems,
over and over we go,
reliving the last few moments.

Stepping into a past remote,
once I had jumped onto
a commuter train, subway, bus seat,
all in a day's work in urban life.

Hitchhiker with a multi-pass,
luring me into the 7 million thicket
faces, hands, fingers, grabbing a handrail---
Into the labor forced on a timeline
not a second to lose, we crammed.

Suddenly, abruptly condensed---
Into a pinpoint. Lockdown. Tomorrow.

5

Unwinding

Freewheeling shopping list

Red beans, lentils, chick peas (organic)
Red rice, brown rice, white rice (organic)
Oatmeal, quinoa,
Milk, butter, yogurt (check dates)
Nutmeg, cinnamon,
Turmeric, ginger (double up)
Sardines, tuna, more sardines
Potatoes, sweet potatoes, squash (lasting)
Apples, bananas, lemons
Bleach, gloves, sponges
Leaks, bell peppers,
Flax seeds, spirulina, tofu (jar)
Checking expiration dates
I am expired first 24 hours
Coffee (organic) shelves are empty?
Strawberries, kiwis, oranges.

Finally, almost forgot:
Toilet paper (4 packs).
Giant packs of 100 for car owners.
My shopping cart has two wheels,
like Grandma's cart, a long time ago...

6

Unravelling

Somber parents, playful babes, nervous teens?

Passing each other,
brimming over, my shopping cart drags,
drooping bags of toilet paper,
and a backpack packed
with essentials?

Reversing the mind to family lore,
depression days moulded Grandpa,
rotating pantry to keep updated, even
50 years on, he prepared for the worse.

I am preparing for the unknown...
Bubonic plague or financial ruin,
None of the above, all of the above.

Mothers' faces pass me on the walk home,
hiding the reality, shifting eyes

scanning my heavy load, up and down
rethinking their strategy? A few bags...

Children skipping along,
no school tomorrow,
teens sticking close,
near Mama,
strange,
only family
groups,
on these sidewalks.

Or solitary ones
Like I, the poet.

7

Goose Down to Lock-Down,

Mother Goose lays her first eggs at sunset.
I had been strolling all winter, most afternoons, in my new locale outside Madrid. A small town on a commuter route. I was refreshed by the flow of the river, a cacophony of sounds. It rekindled a childhood, dreamy sort of hobby; bird watching. With gifted binoculars, I nonchalantly observed migrations overhead, nest building rituals and waterfowl skimming. A canvas of color with rotating blossoms. Finally, the first delicate eggs appeared on goose island.

Timeless less less
Clocks tick not tock

It never dawns on you,
Meaningless time.

Time is of the essence, really?
clock began to tick.

In the first day of *"No School"*
traffic was nullified,
seemed like we
were in a slow motion
time frame, stuck in a projector.

Skidding to a stop,
the train driver halts,
tries to avoid an obstacle
on the tracks, too late?

Here the tracks disappeared
destinations were merged into ONE.

We were getting off midstream,
streamlining time into a single day.

Day 1, then Day 2, the clock ticked
No teen age chatter, rather
joining their family groups
keeping distance, from
lonely geriatrics, singles, runners,
afternoon walks with eyes diverted
in a Latin country, a foreign language.

Fishermen celebrated with laughter
Catching carp at the end of a lazy day.

All in a timeless march, March 2020.

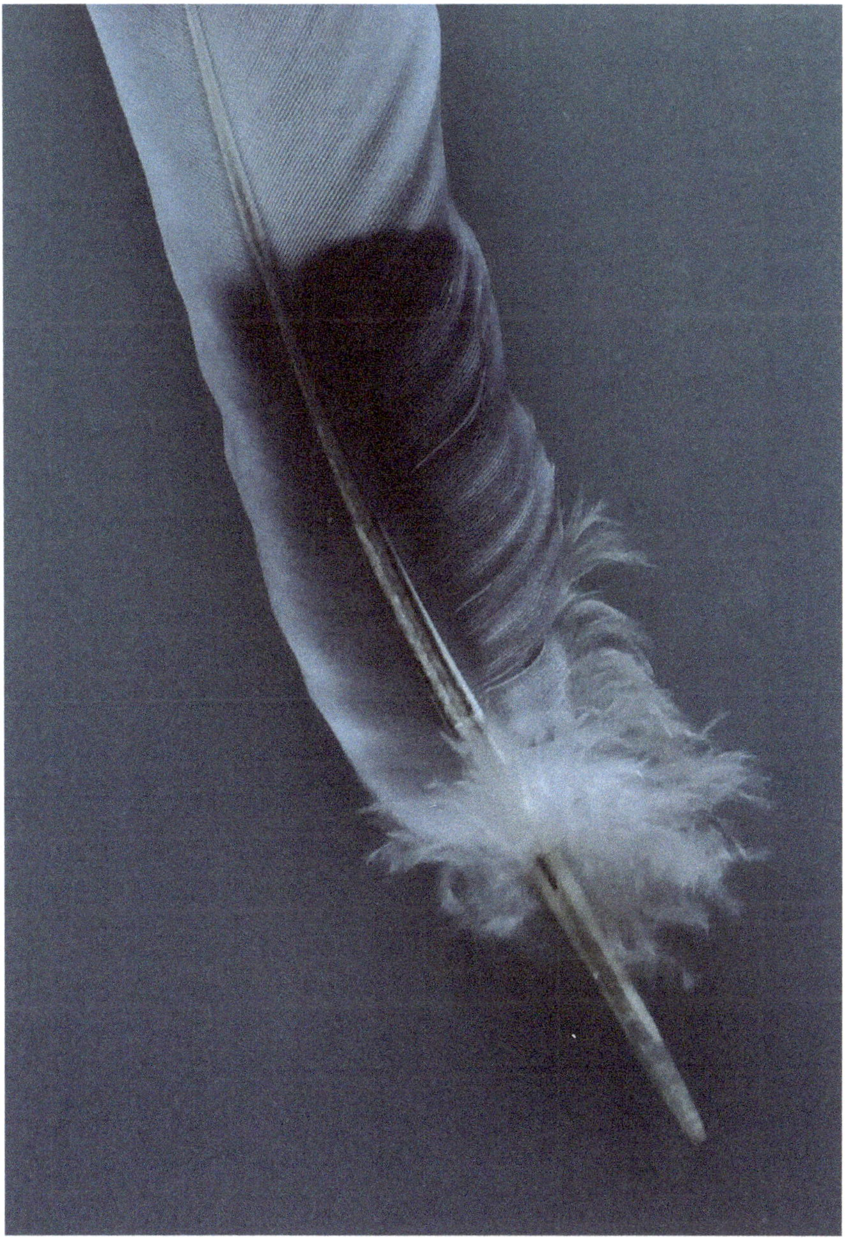

Goose Down Quill
R. Ruiz Scarfuto 2020

8

12 Days of Quarantine

Where am I gonna put all these red beans and rice for a Monday night?

On the first day, pack rat skills emerge
Big 5 questions: Where, where...where?

To figure out
the puzzle of putting away
the freewheeling shopping list

Red beans, lentils, chick peas (start soak)
Red rice, brown rice, white rice (3 kinds?)

Oatmeal, quinoa, (not enough)
raisins, walnuts, almonds, cranberries.
milk, butter, yogurts (why some many?)

My kitchen counter
now a spice island
rosemary, thyme, oregano,
cinnamon, nutmeg, vanilla,
cumin, coriander, black pepper,
turmeric, ginger, garlic.

Where's the garlic?
Tomorrow, I am too tired.

Sardines, tuna, more...[repeat] smelley
one potato 2 sweet potatoes, squash
apples, bananas, lemons,
leaks, peppers, cabbage.

New fridge rocks out, just in time!

Coffee (maybe not enough, ooops)
Strawberries, kiwis, oranges (good deal)
4 packs of toilet paper (hope it's enough)

And the partridge in a *spare* tree.

9

Me & The Cube: Be-tween

Cubism, Surrealism? This is Realism

Picasso explored the art of cubism,
romantic idea in Paris in an artist bubble,
moving on to surrealism with Dali,
I am here trying to wrap my mind,
around the 4 walls that will be my cube,

It was all surreal and yet so REAL.

How did we get here so quick?
just the other day we were celebrating;
March 8th Women's Day around the globe,
except Italy, I thought that was strange?
I was told they couldn't go outside.

Madrileños now
on the same path;
gorgeous sunny day,
trapped in a cube.

Ice cube, distant, cold
new era Madrid,
shocking photos,
of empty streets,
in an ex-vibrant city,
paralyzed in shock.

Anxiety begins
to set in
Surrealism
overtakes
Cubism,
$E=MC^2$
cubed in,
Realism.

We are
in for
a long
-haul
flight,

Be-
tween
walls

Alone.

10

Fever Weaver

Spring weather has arrived in Madrid. I am out enjoying the sun!

When I first arrived in Madrid, the people (Madrileños) commented that they were flexible due to the weather. The change in seasons can be drastic from cold with bits of snow in winter to hot like an oven in summer. Spring had its ups and downs, week to week, day to day. If it were a sunny day in spring, everyone was out in short sleeves enjoying the change. However, the quick fluctuations easily brought about colds and fevers.

No one wants to admit it

Me, fever, no.
No, fever, for me.
Weaving back and forth
Between yes, maybe, no
Nonononone
I gave in to the thermometer.

Not one, but two
Try the old one, 96.8 normal (F)
It that 98? Wait
Try the new one, 36.7 normal (C)
It reads 38? Too late.

So much for assuming.
Game changer.
I'm self-quarantined
Confined at will, willingly,
Safe for others
Am I safe?
I ask ...me, myself and I
No one answers.
I am a host now
Who is this house guest, anyway...?

Aspirin to the rescue?

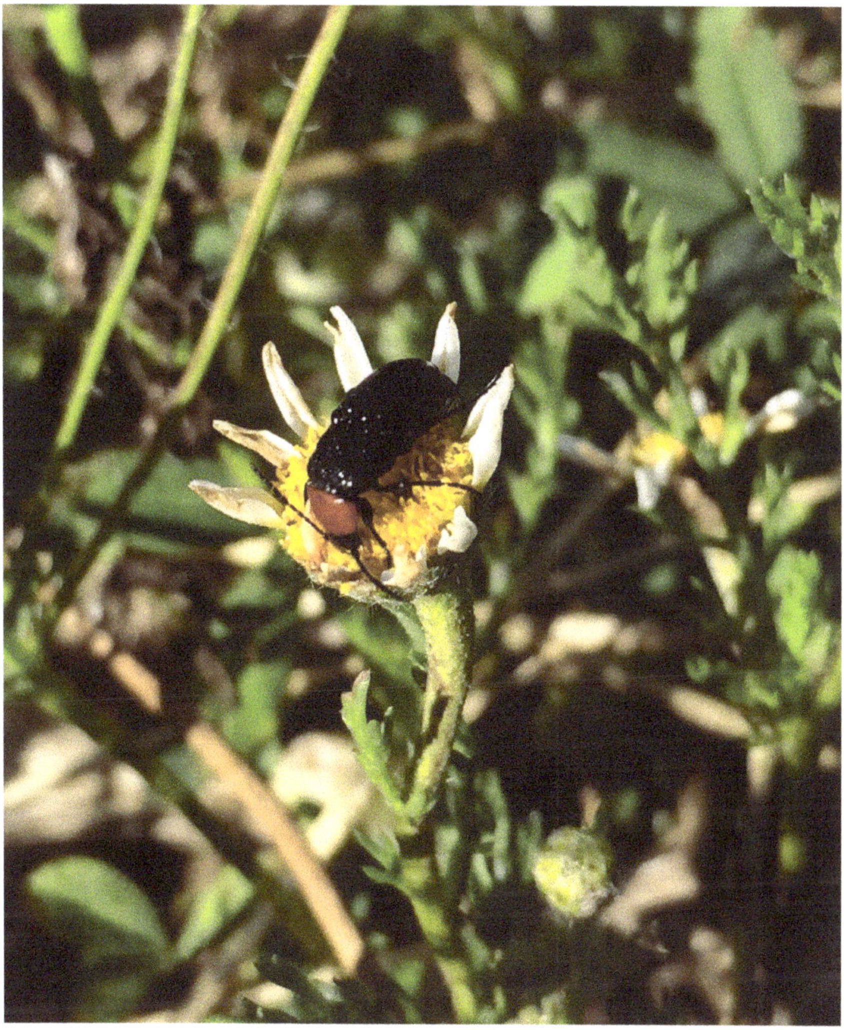

R. Ruiz Scarfuto 2020

11

I can do this! Round 1

Hopscotch choices are a child's,
illness choices are adult's,
medicine and remedies are individual,
based on past experience and body fluids.

For me, it's been a bit of aspirin with food,
takes down the fever, and off we go
To work, to work, and overwork.

Never really questioned it.

Alert comes in,
"Do not take aspirin"
Ride out the fever,
Build up your forces
Makes sense, I'll do it.

Choices from the outset,
change the outcome.

Round 1, the bell sounds
fever has a head start.
"Ready or not, here I come"

Suddenly I am fighting,
in the heavyweights,
I can do this!

12

Who was I kidding?

Round 2: Liar Liar Pants on Fire Baby!

Once you see
the shore slipping away
a journey really begins,
to unknown seas.

I only had three aspirins in the house,
already decided to fight it out,
hid those tablets in the junk drawer.
Sometimes you just gotta fool yourself,
Be strong, hold out, get tough.

I have been alone in Hong Kong,
On the 18th floor of Chung King Mansion,
Lying in a youth hostel dorm
Sick with diarrhoea, lonely,
Reading *Papillon* to pass the time,
I can do this, low fever, no problem...

Breakfast with ginger tea & toast (no coffee)
I am so cold! Warming, soothing, spices, relief!
Suddenly I am exhausted at 9:30 am?
I go lay my head down,
on my pillow,
I doze off lightly,
kinda nice for a change.

Only to be woken up,
to a house party,
in my kidneys,
burn baby burn! OUCH!
Round 2, fever wins.

13

Dish Drain, Energy Drain

New dishware delights for housewarming.
A few weeks before lockdown, I went to buy a ladder. While shopping, I was distracted by some lovely plates on sale. My favorite color; sea foam, light turquoise. I splurged to create a novel décor in my newly settled kitchen. I was thinking of guests for tea, so I opted for matching tea mugs, place mats and appetizer tray. I was drawn to a set of nice sharp knives to replace the dull ones. Finally, out of the corner of my eye, I spotted a chopping block.

Tortoise Turn: Hiding out in the shell

Turtles have got the ideal retreat center,
I am locked away in my shell,
Under siege from this awful calamity,
One long standing head ACHE!
Unquenchable cellular screams (WATER)
Dunking liters of liquidity into a vacuum.

How come I haven't had a bathroom run?

Stomach empties in toilet bowl,
Even with little smell faculties,
a stench fumes, upsetting even Me!

Tucked into bed, in my turtle shell,
No comfort for the excruciating limbs,
Grin, bear, it and check for chatting jokes.
Hibernation mode turns over to sleep.

Who's gonna cook? My turn again.
Slacking to the kitchen, facing the chopping block,
One slice at a time, takes all MIND
Good I have that Buddhist meditation practice,
To draw on, empty mind, so boggled
Careful don't cut your finger, no hospitals!

Boil the water, drop in chunks, wait
I can hardly stand UP, sit down
Sipping SOUP (turtle slow motion) .

Fever 24/7

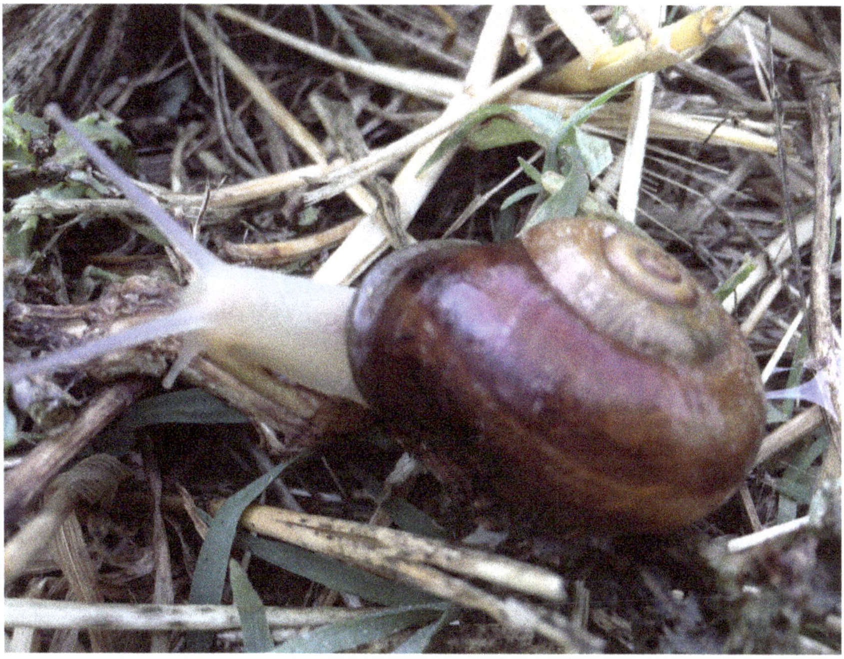

Snail's Retreat

R. Ruiz Scarfuto 2020

14

Saturday Night Fever, Fever

Saturday Night Fever, hangs over Sun-Day blues

Sleep day? Sleep night?
Pain seizes to amaze my kidneys,
Lymph node overload,
Legs are rest-less-not,
Dancing in the middle of the night,
Getting used to a new "feeling" inside.

Shake and bake this body,
I am not giving in to you!
Virus weaving in and out of my organs,
Plasma, bone marrow, digestive tract,
Low grade heat, high voltage pain!

Sprawled on couch, limp
Suddenly phone rings,
distraction, good!
Red Cross! Perfect, to the rescue
What? donation?

I thought it was to inquire,
about my condition.
Brain is mushy,
I say, "Call me back in 14 days"
Hesitant response...script ends..."ok"

Back to my hangover,
from Saturday night
dancing with fever, fever,
passing the baton
Sun-Day blues.

15

Monday-Mundane

Weekend Overrated

Mondays are never my favorites,
Lyrical melodies drum it in from early age,
"Rainy days and Mondays..."
"Monday/Monday"

Not this Monday, I was looking forward
To the weekend being OVER!

Not so lucky, lingering into Day 4.
Fever hides out somewhere,
In the bedding! Gotta wash it out!

What a drag...drag off the sheets,
Drag them down the hall,
Drag out the washing liquid
Wait to drag them out and hang.

Meanwhile chop the soup contents,
Meander to dreaded dirty sink,
Who's afraid of dishes? Me...

Siesta time, 3pm.
Sirens whistle outside.

Is it time to clap for medical staff?
Now it's 8pm!

Day gone...sunset falling down
Good news; clean sheets!
Is it Tuesday, yet?

16

Daydreams I

My first daydreams transported me across the sea.
As a child, I liked to jump in the sea foam of the Pacific Ocean. On the shore, I frolicked in the tidepools, fascinated by sea life. At sunset my imagination melted into the horizon. I drifted into a daydream, across the Sea. Albeit, our sunsets in L.A. were polluted, psychedelic experiences; bar none. By the age of 21, I was on a plane to Japan without a clue of how I got there or what I would find. It was a magical trip that changed my life.

Daylight Haze, Brain Waves Wave Good-Bye

Into the Ocean, I dive to the unknown,
Under the waves, where coral lives, calmly
Tropical fish swim near, tiny bubbles a-bound...

I am in their dream,
twilight hues,
twilight moves,
twilight soothes...

Serenading my five senses,
Open to the 6th,
pulsating colors
reflected by sunrays
I see the surface of water
Ebbing and flowing over head.

Life on the shore, continues
never-the-less,
I am here in Everland,
hours pass over me,
a ripple in time,
1,000 per/hour
reduces down to...
an hour, a minute, an instant, ONE.

Sea-time is Goddess time.

I tumble deeper,
into the sway,
of the sea grass tune.

As I go,
an invisible presence
guides me
by the hand,
I can no longer resist,
the force
of the swell,
I let go
of the fishing line

I am alone
in a familiar place.

Where am I?
(querying innocently)
I see the shore
distorted.

Me in the arms
in HER arms way
en-gulfed by the Sea.

I am barely awake
I am bare.

17

Cosmic Breath

Unveiling OM
"You call me, I call you."

I call upon the Cosmos
for comfort.

A humpback whale appears!

In my mind, I call Ommm
I am not sleeping, but I am vigilant...
My inner ear vibrates, OMMM

Through the song of the humpback
I send out my call again "om om"
Faint sounds of an Angelic "OM, OM"
Swirl on the current,
coming closer and closer
I feel Prana arriving.

I inhale, my gills fill up
with HER life force
Cosmic breath.

Humpback dives deeper; winking at me
I fall into a deeper daydream
vision now blurred,
I lost sight of the tail
of my Humpback friend,
I can only follow its song.

Fused with the "OM OM OM"
I repeat in my mind, "om om om"
I feel a soft veil brush up against my face,
energy changes, where am I now?

18

Pro-found Fathoms of the Sea

Cracks in the Sea are like cracks in your Heart;
Hidden until you reach bottom.

Fathoms beneath my bed,
Covers blanket my existence,
I am here more hours in a day, than not.

I drop through a gap, into a trench
Beneath reality, surreal, profound
Low levels of oxygen to my brain
Allow me to enter an altered state.

Consciousness rules, begin to separate,
Once beyond the veil, Maya, has less grip
I am not in her world anymore,
Wordy, worldly ties fray, meaning-less

I am fully in OM,
HER vibrations re-sound,
I enter the sacred passage,
Overriding all worlds on shore,
I am in the Heart of our planet.

Here in the fathoms of the Sea,
I am stunned with HER essence,
inner and outer, no boundries
between Sea and shore,
I have found a rare place,
to pirouette, to dance.

Beauty once concealed,
offers to become
my Cosmic companion.
her True Self,
bestowed in my heart.

My prayers
are answered,
I accept.

19

Beauty rides on back of Cosmic Breath

My first snow was on a lotus pond;
snowflakes descended from Heaven.

I found myself with a view of a lotus pond in Japan for the summer. Autumn came and maple trees wore golden robes. Nothing mystified me, up until winter. I had not known snow country. I was awakened ever so lightly by an interloper. The sound of snow, delicate to ears and eyes. I witnessed a glimpse of Beauty that morning. She tapped on my heart, engraved her seal. It was lodged deep inside, waiting to be retrieved one day.

Unintentional delay in breath chisels my stone away.

My breath is slower and slower,
Movement follows behind in step,
I am out of control of my material world,
Lungs respire fewer strokes of genius,

I no longer abide by concrete equations,
I surrender to the Cosmic breath...

BEAUTY reigns in this profound chasm,
She rules the game and I don't mind,
My weary body surrenders to HER wisdom,
Like a gong that vibrates longer in open spaces,
I am open to the Goddess that re-verberates
Speaks with no words, that I can decipher.

My soul tells me, to allow HER, to hold me,
In peace, *unfathomed* in waking hours,
I am not asleep, but in a new awakening,
I cherish this grace granted to me,
even if I have to breathe, slower/slower.

Stone dissolves by rain,
ever so slowly,
I feel the dust,
falling
off.

20

Rain tapping on the door to my Soul

Rain and I intermingle at the window/pane;
In my own/pain I am gifted a long lost treasure.

Tap Tap Tap ever so lightly,
You visit me like an angel,
on my windowpane.

We are separated by a thin sheathe,
I am aware and yet unaware.
White lace curtains
mist my view.

teardrop sonata,
fuses you (*rain*) with my state,

Entranced by the rolling
of droplets,

Unhurriedly
rippling,
from place
to place.

I am the sole
witness of this ballet,
delicate...
as slow
as my heart
beat...

Rain across the window-pane
Yearning to meet its destination.

To unhinge, wither, the stone door to my Soul.

Only in this agony of slowness, breath/less
I am reduced to a rambling,
as pure as a raindrop.

"Open your heart" says the Yogi master
All those years,
I never asked "*how?*"

21

Mind-less matter banished from my constellation

Milky way hurls me forward;
Law of attraction carries me to the edge.
Stone door crumbles silently behind me,
I am inside my milky hollow envelope.
Outside world is a swishing babble,
all/though news attempts to bite my ear.
My core is deep inside itself,
Turned off/inside/out/side/down.
Tower of babble, like the tower of Pisa,
I was leaning towards untainted BEAUTY,
Unlike the current outside, in real-time.

In this secluded gallery, of my own atrium,
attention to the lushness of inert colours,
hurls me forward into a milky way spin.

Peacock blues grace through the grass,
flamingo pinks appear on lotus petals,
immortal - truthful pigments, appear as
eternal transparency, across the spectrum.

BEAUTY has come to retrieve her gift,
after trials and tribulations,
breaking the seal she left behind, on my heart,
near a lotus pond, long ago.
SHE pulls out the treasure, from its sacred place.

A new dawn pivoting on twilight's toes,
there is Silence; no light, no dark.
SHE places it in front of me.

I feel the links of a neck-lace clasp,
We are joined, we are O-N-E.
my heart is OPEN.

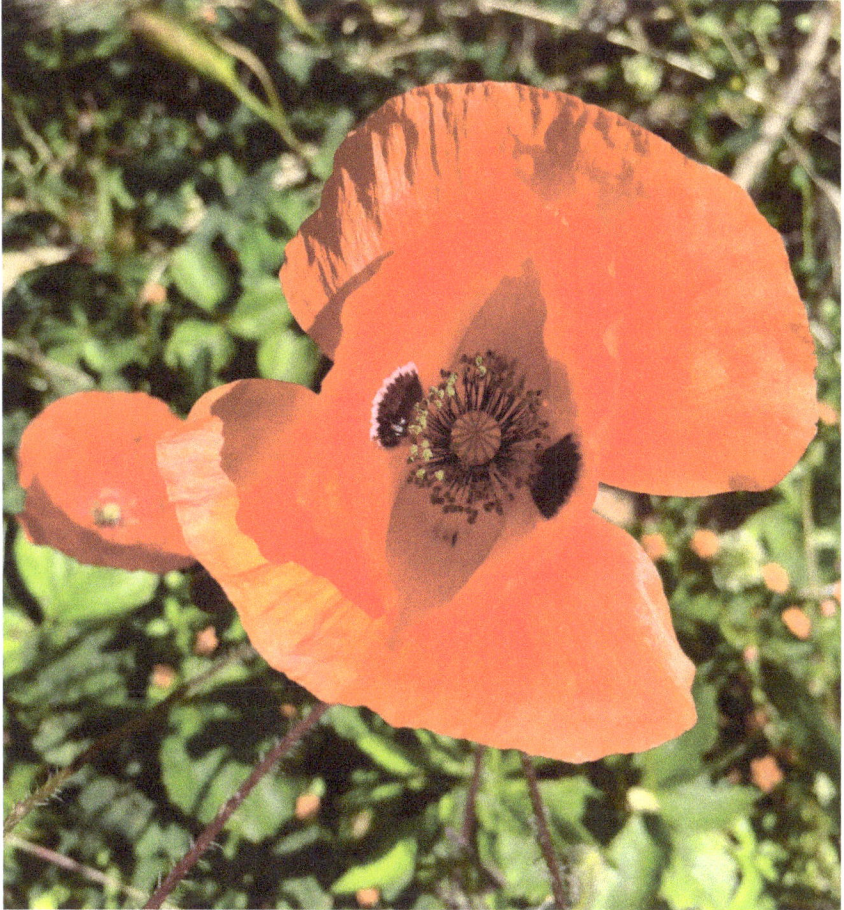

Heart of the Poppy
R. Ruiz Scarfuto 2020

22

Who left the window open in my lungs?

I used to come home from school and say "today's a really smoggy day." I knew it because my lungs ached. Next day, the news would announce "high alert." That meant no going outside to play. Earthquakes, wild-fires, tumble weeds, bear attacks, tarantulas and rattlesnakes are just a few of my vague memories of wild life in California. All have a story of first times. However, smog was just part of the overall picture and your lungs hurt more in summer.

Isolation erases your "common" sense.

Signs of Covid 19 narrowed down,
To sound bites, panic buttons flare,
Fever and shortness of breath! Not me!
Run to the doctor, better yet the hospital.

Overloaded doctor doors,
Revolving in my head,

Emergency; no rooms available,
It's time to put your big boots on,
Stay home and isolate, mate.

If I could just stay away from the hospital,
I would be a forsaken winner, but happy.
Formula 1, race to keep it together.

After the fever subsided, kidneys calmed,
Legs took their turn tormenting my sleep,
Gotta do a lymph scrub, lonely chore,
Relief at last! Quiet slumber.

Then came the strange sensation:
Who left the window open in my lungs?

23

Santa Ana Winds visit my deserted window

Prickly tumble weeds amass inside my lungs, disturbing.

Wheezing is dubbed "shortness of breath"
Perhaps I was confused, not me? Winded maybe.
Less oxygen leaves dust on the brain.

An eerie hissing, on each inhalation, breathtaking in fact?
A cunning uprising to take over the homestead.
Finally, I plotted to hide behind a fence, lay low.

Just slouch in bed,
like a slacker (novel approach)

My mind reflected,
on black and white cinema,

Sick people stayed in bed,
with comforting pillows.
Others waited on them,
with soup, not here.

Chores to do,
soup to cook,
dishes to wash,
and only then,
was I free to crash in bed,
waiting for nothing, really.

I forwent even yoga,
at this point-
pathetic, anyway.

No one came,
to close the window.
Gusting wind blows,
through my ribs,
no deep breaths for me.

I could only wait it out,
like a sentinel on watch,
of an unknown enemy.

24

Moon waning, I'm gasping, who's watching?

Balancing act on a swaying tight rope;
All on my own in space and time.

How are you today? Came the messages,
"Bit better" my dry, short response,
For days, and days, and days...
Lost count of the never-ending story.

Behind the iron curtain,
Mineral supplies losing ground,
Red blood, white blood, all cells zapped!

I counter with ancient Ayurveda teas
Boiled up bitter, copper turmeric roots.

Cut with a tangy ginger splash.
Don't forget the spicy black pepper, just a dash.
Garlic, coriander and lots of
'Love"
Says the Yogi Master.

"Keep laughing,"
says a spirit from far above.

Food for thought,
you are what you eat,
Mind, body and soul complete.

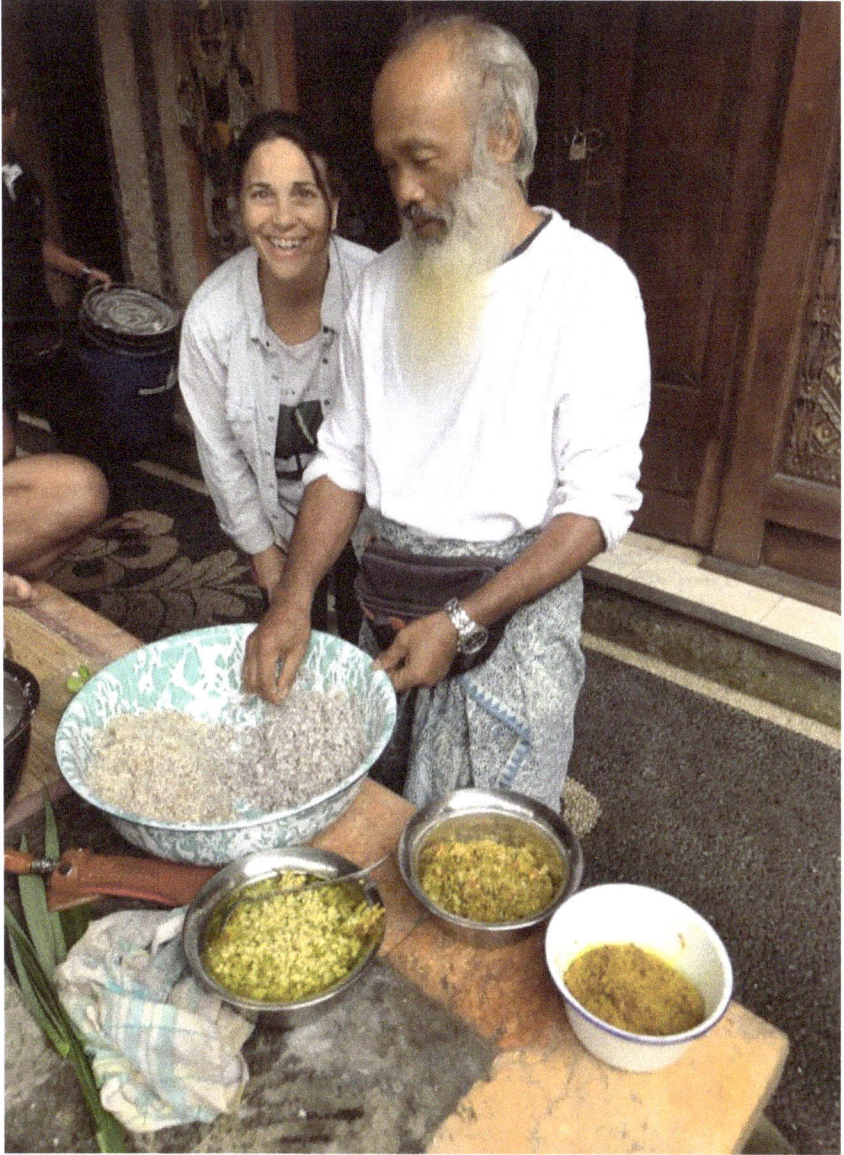

Cooking with the Yogi Master
Rosalinda Ruiz Scarfuto 2019, Bali

25

Neighborly love in a dystopian utopia

I grew up with friendly neighbors that are now life-long friends. Every country has its cultural boundaries. Some talk, some listen, some do both. "Love your neighbor" famous quote from a prophet. My neighbors from childhood shared a space for playing, celebrating, and growing together. We needn't dress up, just hanging out. I missed them as I travelled across the globe. Nevertheless, I found other neighbors to bond, in new and different ways. Some became friends and were added to my good vibe tribe.

Sounds of silence abound
with spurts of routine rattle.

Strange how silence,
takes over a pandemic,
movements are deliberate,
streets abandoned.

Neighbors on the other hand, persevere
Carrying on, coping in community.

Side by side in a soft routine,
I barely knew any of these folks.

Suddenly I got to know them, all at once,
from a hole in the wall, 101 apart-ments.
An immense patio, bound us together.
We hung laundry together,
cooked together,
and listened.

A violin player practiced, 5pm sharp,
Sisters giggled just before lunch, everyday,
Feet pounded at 7pm, on the exercise wheel.

All followed by gapping hours of silence,
boredom I suppose for them, soothing to me.

Silence became the new norm, in dystopia,
Neighborly love as I see it, utopia for the ill.

26

Doctor, Doctor tell me what you know at the eye of the storm!

Never flinching, she is my heroine, Dr. María Jesús.

When no one had extra time, at the peak of the curve,
Dr. María Jesús, tapped in a text to me.

I held on to these words,
Falling off the hem of her medical gown,
Like clutching Mama's apron strings, to shelter me, in place.

She traded in her surgeon tools,
to take on overflow calls,
lonely desk job.

Following patients into the night,

on the paper trail, she weathered the storm.
I was another one, of thousands of cases,
avoiding collapsing lungs, a hospital bed.

It came down to the small print,
on my cell phone screen
from Dr. MJ.
Transmitting assurance,
unbeknownst to me,
I stayed calm,
storm passed over.

I am utterly grateful,
her attention to details, lifting me,
to some kind of normal.

How can a few words of confidence,
boost the immune? You ask?
Change the mood of a patient?
Change their destination papers.

I slowly got better,
no hospital for me,
no nightmares to face.

Dr. MJ rejoiced,
in her own quiet way):
surely she had many more calls
to chase, at her lonely desk.

27

It takes a tribe: create a ritual for daily bread

Sunrise to sunset: LOL (lots of love and laughs)

I called on my tribe, to keep myself sane,
in other words chatting.

My days were flanked by
"Buenos Dias" & "Buenas Noches"
"Good Morning" & "Good Night"

I could hardly read
long, political, winded, chats
Let alone books of opinions.
(how to did they fit it all in?...*read more*)

“Please no more conspiracy speeches,”
exhausted by virus invasion,
I begged, "This is REAL!"

I veered toward the absurd,
and comedy central,
“More jokes please!”
they cured cancer in the 70’s,
laughing it away? Right?

Laughter in isolation,
is an inside joke,
lonely on the couch,
but chuckling with my tribe,
did relieve the pain...
kept me sane.

I feasted on this daily bread,
a chain, chatting ritual,
a constant in the chaos.

To be inspired and To inspire

with a forward button,
on our fingertips.

My tribe laughed
me through,
the bluest hours
the longest days,
weeks, a month
and more...

I began to type
in French,
Italian, Japanese,
even Australian,
“hey mate”

Latest in from Zimbabwe,
“just starting lockdown"
"how are you?”

Boat was bigger,
than Noah’s ark
on a good day.

all
in it,
together,
some jumping off,
others climbing on... LOL

28

Silent Spring 2020: Bird calls thrive in the void!

Walking to school in Spring, meant enjoying the high, green clover. Lasting memories in a land mostly brown and dry, near the Mohave desert. Running free, creating trails in open fields was especially rewarding in Spring. Hiding and seeking nothing special. Nightly owls haunted me at bedtime, but pigeons gleefully greeted me at dawn. Memoirs hard to erase. I did miss the howl of owls, when they cut down the trees.

Blackbird Singing in the Day: Nature Alarming us!
(sweeter than any phone tweet)

"Wake up humans!" "*Calling all birds of a feather"*
"To flock together," Blackbird yodels at 5 am!
Silent airways in lockdown, leave room for an echo
Symphony of nature, filling the void.

Sweet sound reaching my bed,
at the break of dawn,
Beats the humdrum of diesel trucks,
wheeling under my window.

A twist on the theme,
Silent Spring, in the 60's,
When a woman noticed,
birds songs disappearing.

How fragrant the sound,
of this amazing grace.
Just outside to pals,
they chant "hello" "where are you?"
Taking back the daybreak!
Me, cheering them on.

Young swallows chirping,
for their morsels to come,
under terracotta eves,
in abondoned bull ring.

Sunrise has risen,
Nature has spoken first, today.
I pull back the covers,
rise to the occasion,
It keeps me alive! Inspired!
To begin again!

I peer into the indigo sky,
from my living room terrace,
"I'm here, your human pal"
No yodeling, yet.

29

My closest companions: radish tops and mustard seeds

Mini organic garden sprouts up,
and whispers in my ear.

How to start a garden in a limited space?
No seeds, no soil, you ask?
In the midst of self-quarantine,
with no place to go, fresh greens running low,
plagued by an insatiable thirst,
fridge looking quite bare, I saw the colors
of my stockpile, eroding away.
radish tops, carrot greens, why not plant these?
I once saw a video, got nothing to lose.

Standing at the chopping block,
an epiphany from Heaven! Save the Seeds!
Green peppers, pumpkin seeds (roast or plant?)
Apple and lemon seeds? Who knows?
It was like panning for gold, nuggets in the bank!

I began to set up a drying station,
recycled planters, milk cartons, cute!
Oops! No soil! Now what?
I had one huge planter with bulbs (waiting to bloom)
two smaller pots; one full, one empty.
I couldn't bare the thought,
of throwing out the daffodil bulbs.
I made do with two half pots,
planted the radish and carrot tops in one,
green pepper seeds in the other.

Sprouts? How about these mustard seeds?
destined for a lymph scrub,
I threw a few in for good luck.
Eureka! I had my mini garden.

As the days dilly-dallied on,
with lockdowns stretching 5 weeks,
6 weeks, on and on...
Still, day by day, I woke up
to greet my mini garden friends,
As I grew stronger, they grew taller.

One day, they whispered,
"Everything's gonna be alright, "stick with us."
Bless us our Lord for these little gifts of joy!

30

Under my balcony: things I saw, things I missed

Street life changes by the hour;
I happened to see less than my neighbor

Dogs, owners, pooping, scooping,
All hours, morning, noon and night
Silently apart, avoiding contact,
Empty buses rolling by, masked drivers
Street sweepers sweeping, here and there
Water trucks slowly refilling supplies, no hurry
Pedestrians destined to destinations, bags in hand (proof)
Mood swings from dull to duller
Weeds growing high and higher
It was my window to the world, albeit a small world.

One day after lockdown, my neighbor proclaims,
shockingly: “Don’t talk to me about football anymore...”
confused, I inquiry, "Que pasa?"
then, he tells me his view
under our balconies:

hour after hour, in procession,
endless hearses rolling silently,
to destinations known,
respective mortuaries,
just over yonder.

What I missed in the back bedroom,
afternoons in bed, laying in wait,
i am sure it was a blessing,
a real downer for anyone,
let alone someone ill, like me.

No sympathy
for the frivolous,
football shut out
to the muteness
of black hearses.
far away from me,
hindsight 2020.

I am so thankful,
for what i missed.

31

Learning to walk again?

My grand-nephew was just learning to walk on my last visit. Cute at the age of a toddler. I had not realized the devastating toll that the virus had taken on my body; robbing my blood cells (red, white and yellow) and then I lost muscle mass. The result was not cute; walking further than the kitchen was tiresome. I had three flights of stairs to battle with grocery bags, and 3 blocks to a market. Venturing out was a big deal. On the upswing, it had devoured fat cells at a record speed. I hit my ideal weight in less than 21 days!

Semi-bedridden for 21 days has its disadvantages;
some more obvious than others.

At 5 weeks, "Still recovering?" they remarked (friends).
Why was that surprising? I wondered?

I vividly
recall the first day,

I thought:
Time for exercise? Can I?
It was a truly
a new notion.

Carefully cautious.
I asked for a recovery
program
from my doctor,
hospitals gave them out
for free in a pdf form.

Strange for merely a fever,
shortness of breath,
aches and pains in the kidneys,
low energy.

I was naïve
to second guess
my body's deficiency.

Revving up
for arms circles,
tiny leg lifts (in a chair)
Mind you,
I couldn't even stand up, to get dressed
I chalked it up to depleted energy.

Simply put,
it was lack
of leg muscles.
down 9 kilos (20 lbs).
3 weeks, too soon.

Abundantly clear, later
as I strolled, awkwardly
to the market, a disconnect;
my legs in mutiny,
against my brain,
what a weird sensation,
Am I imagining this?
I was suddenly 95,
and needed a walker?

None of this recovery
was cute...
cumbersome, yes.

Taking it slow,
taking my time,
not at the pace
of the world clock.

32

Stuck between a rock lung, a hard heart?

Asking for help with my heart, "Fire breathing" "push it out!" replies the Yogi master. *Really?*

Take a ride on,
the rollercoaster rebound,
Novel, novel, novel ups
and downs,
never the same!
Watch out for rare sensation,
approaching inside
the left lung.

What's that?
A cramp in my heart?
Mind racing to worse scenario,
After all this homecare,

Do I need a hospital?

Normal, says the doctor...
pressure on the heart
I turned to the yogi master,
what's good for the heart?

Me, in panic,
slow down...it's the heart!

Don't be stupid.

I consult for gentle yoga
to relax, maybe?

Yogi master prescribes,
a mighty aerobic
yoga program,
"Do it fast,
and breathe loud
from your mouth"

You're kidding?
Fast and hard?

"Yes!" (was the comeback)

Time for fire
breathing (Bhastika)
Time to push, beyond
my common sense.

Prana, Prana, Prana Yama
Om Shanti Shanti Shanti OM!

33

Out & About; Phase Zero

I can hardly believe it or not?
Look I'm outside on my bike, and you?
Fresh air, a long-lost commodity,
surged in Spring of 2020.

While others slumped,
in the silence
of the low market demand
Pollution lockdown,
skies turned blue, a breather at last!

I am riding my bike,
almost swooning with joy!

Today, May 2, 2020
we flattened the curve.

Unforgettable flash,
shared by all,
May 2nd Goya's time,
Madrid defeated
Napoleon troops,
farmers no less.

Swerving back and forth on two wheels,
out & about, on a tree-lined road.
Nothing like country morning air,
crisp cascades of sun rays, a robust moment.

Goose island full of gawking geese,
"Surprise we're back!" No pausing today.
I rode, and rode as far as my lungs
could go and time permitted.

New normal, outdoor activities regulated to protect,
06-10 am, at the starting gate, 14-69 year olds,
10-12 noon, strolling, 70+ group
12-7 pm, final stretch, kids under 14+caregivers,
7-11pm, 14-69 group, second chance, repeat.
All day, all night, birds, squirrels, geese,
free to sing and chirp for us, in-spiration.

I relished the break,
from essential tasks,
wilderness on my tongue,
against the wind.

Capturing this instant,
a Selfie, click, send.
City folks pay attention,
to open space, behind me.

Gone was my norm,
of urban touting,
droves confined,
to the contours of asphalt.

Country life
never felt so right,
I was truly outside
the city scape,
what a relief,
AHHA!

34

Passing trains, a blip in my peripheral vision

I will never forget the day I took a walk on a country road. I found myself beneath elegant storks flying low overhead as they landed to feast in the rows of alfalfa. Sweet smell of fresh cut fields in the morning mist as I witnessed the sunrise; a piece of heaven. I rented a plot of land for a whole-hearted recovery; seedlings, sunshine and old fashion sweat. I would be tilling the soil, planting a dream and forgetting Madrid.

I have even forgotten the train schedule;
Let bygones be bygones.

Before, I saw the countryside
zoom by from a train,
now from this perspective, in a silent field
trains whizz by like a toxic sneeze.

No matter how comfortable the seats,
on the bullet train, faster than lightening,
I preferred the grounded, sodden seat
on this tiny piece of Earth;
the hearth of life.

Moving at the speed of a sun dial,
at the pulse of our breath,
here in the garden,
side by side with seedlings,
growing in the moonlight,
surprising us at dawn.

Picking wild roses,
strawberries and figs,
nourishing a forgotten palette
restimulating my sense of smell.

Wondering when the peacocks
will ever stop wailing
louder than anything around,
even feline fights.

I hear the rails squeal
and I know train's a coming
bringing home commuters,
like me in a past life.

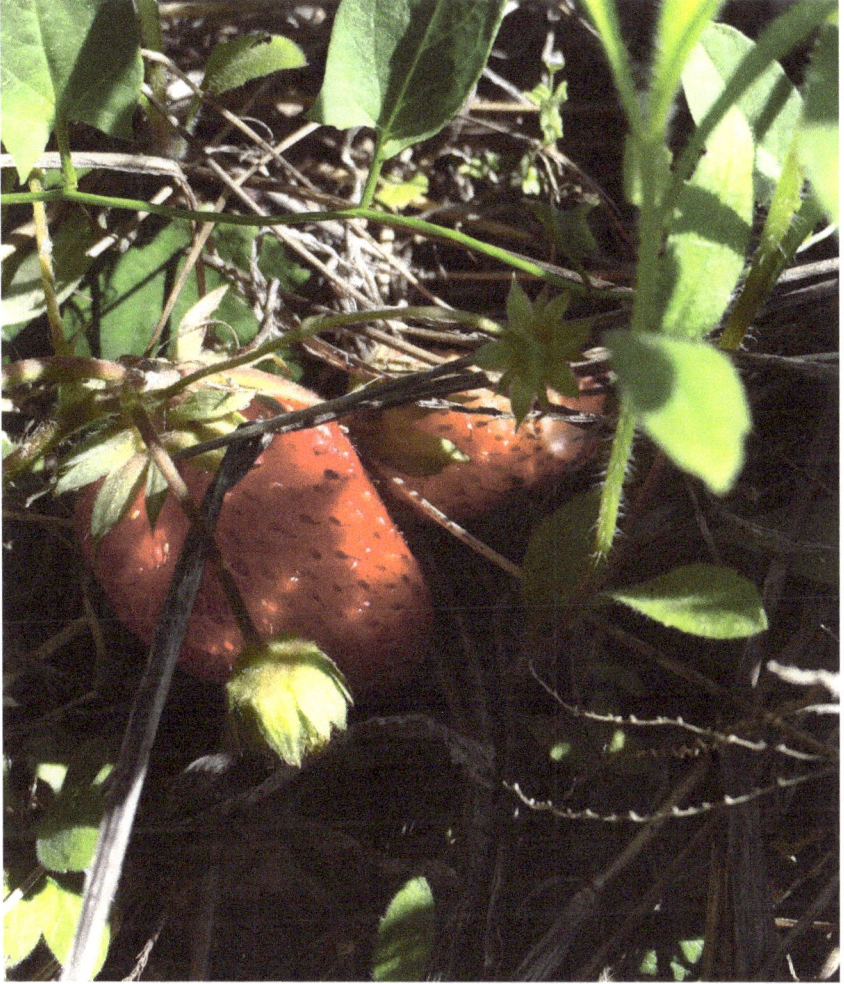

Hide and Seek Strawberries

R. Ruiz Scarfuto 2020

35

San Isidro Bring Us Rain on the Plains in Spain

**I find myself bordering on La Mancha;
Don Quixote and his farmers' wisdom.**

May 15th is St. San Isidro day,
bringing festivities and rain
If you plant too late,
you risk ruin, with a downpour
Quarantine squandered our time,
many planted late.

I ended up so late, I missed the rain,
I planted May 17th,
and saved my seedlings,
thank goodness for that...

My neighbor lost half his garden,
with a sudden downpour, Oh San Isidro!
beginners luck I suppose, first hurdle passed

Moles plagued the fields,
vigilant cats, watchful over burrows
hand fed by Margarita,
frustrated farmers,
dangling their beer bottles
on iron rods, vibrating underground
to show a presence
jiggling, wiggling,
scaring them away in the night.
I would let them be, hoping for harmony.

In the beginning,
I was up to my knees
in horse apples,
planting like crazy,
foraging for reeds
in nearby canals,
whacking at a slant,
bundling them
transforming them
into trellises,
tying up tomatoes,
guiding cucumbers vines.

Prune the melons or not?
Sunflowers sprouting,
peppers plants, dancing with the wind,

Zucchini flowers
appear overnight,
time for pollinatation,
hoping for bees,
farmers wonder if
too many male flowers
not enough females
time to learn basics,
Which one is female?

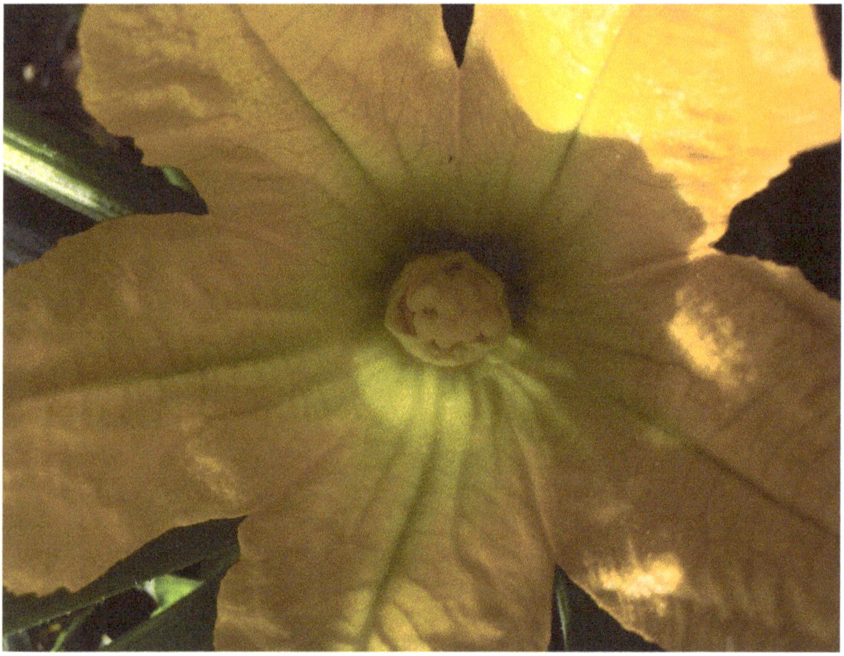

Zucchini Sunrise

R. Ruiz Scarfuto 2020

36

Under the Grape Vine with Lazy Lavender

Grapevine Shade

Shredded, twisted
solid, rooted, winded
matted charcoal trunk.

Grape leaves, dangling
fresh, springy
rough touch,
optical illusion.

Budding fruits,
hang over head,
waiting like me
for sundown breeze.

Lazy Lavender
She invites you to join
in her essence,
Peace—and languid lavender days.

Sun passes now,
moving on to after/noon
humble and perfumed lavender,
purpula—tea, lavishing
into the twilight, moon
shadow of a grapevine
hovers overhead.

37

Butterfly Bliss

Luminous Wings
Lead Me
Home

Fleeting—zig zagging
on this new moon.

22 May, 2020
Calm, serene.
Phase zero.
Ending on a good note

butterflies
frolicking
nectar to nectar.

Oblivious
to our
dilemma.

we lag
behind
mariposa

on her path
light not heavy
the road not taken
our bliss forgotten bliss.

R.

38

What I learned

Introduction

This journey through my body, mind and soul during the coronavirus lockdown came as a surprise to me; hence, I would like to write about its personal impact on me and leave you with some useful hints in dealing with this "novel" virus should it be necessary. In Madrid, people have had various reactions to the virus, from mild to fatal. I fall in the mid-section of this range. Some of my friends had mild versions with flu-like symptoms lasting for approximately a week, with loss of smell and taste (main indicator of Covid-19). I, however, happened to have experienced a full body tour of the virus, with challenges every step of the way. Here in this book, I have attempted to recall the highlights of my illness which I have extracted from my bedside notes written during the 5 weeks with the idea to hopefully help others dealing with the virus. My spiritual practice has evolved from Western to Eastern, with a touch of Native American expressed in respect for the Earth, yoga practice, and love in action. This virus was certainly the "trickster" Coyote pushing me to dig deep to face the Great Spirit; physically, emotionally and spiritually. Ready or not, it was coming, and no hiding. It was like an interior vision quest, rambling through my own organism down to the cellular level. It played with my brain via dehydration and forced me to slow down like a snake in the desert heat. At the worst point, I had no other choice but to give up life as a separate human being in control. I finally fused with Nature, and opened my heart to a new chapter in life.

I understand that you may never come down with Covid-19, but perhaps a loved one will experience the virus. Hopefully, with my account you would be able to understand their symptoms and help them. My intention is to alert the public of the speed of this virus as it attacks the human system, which leaves very little flex time to react. Hence, this book has been created for prevention, fair warning, and hindsight, 2020. I am grateful for information from social media that gave me a sense of the voracity of the virus, which in turn put me on alert from the beginning. One example was the experience explained by a British man in Wuhan recovering from the virus. He had a cold which then moved quickly on to pneumonia, and shortly thereafter he was hospitalized. Considering the impact of his account of the virus, I took all symptoms as serious and any changes as dangerously near the hospital line.

In the beginning I was able to keep up with my meditations and yoga. However, physical yoga was dropped once it was obvious my lungs were debilitated and I needed to stay in bed and be much less active. Nevertheless, I continued meditation sessions of 30 minutes with mantras (singing) and pranayama (breathing) every day to help keep my lungs in minimal shape. I was flustered many days since I could hardly do them, but I continued the practice. At the same time, I was stunned that I could muster up the energy to actually do those sessions, when everything seemed like "mission impossible". Yet the meditation just seemed like food for the soul and essential for my overall well-being. I had to be careful with timing for energy reasons and calculated my food intake ratio to digestion for optimum results. (For example, I had four hours of slow release of energy after eating oatmeal for breakfast).

My mental attitude was vital in keeping everything balanced, and my general knowledge of my body from previous illnesses came in handy. I believe my mindset marked the fine line that separated me from the finish line at home or in a hospital. One can easily spin into a negative spiral, thus weakening the immune system with emotional stress if the mind is left unchecked. I was lucky to have had an early warning from my yoga teacher, who kept me laughing through the first stage. I kept up this attitude by requesting jokes to boost my immune system. Through my WhatsApp contacts I received a constant stream of jokes coming from all angles, with homemade videos and images that seemed endless, along with other messages. I concentrated alone on the lightness of laughter, and it proved to be very effective.

Discipline was another mindset that was vital. It took all my complete attention to keep up a routine (designed to meet each phase). It meant that I use mindfulness to move slowly and stay focused on tasks through each process and adapt to all the changes in my bodily reaction to the virus. Now I am glad I had been trained first from my youth by my strict parents. For the past 25 years that training has been followed up by a yoga master with a strict character. The uniqueness of my yoga teacher is his profound gift for joking when times are tough, like Covid-19, and his positive attitude in confronting health challenges. He also utilizes Ayurveda (ancient Indian medicinal philosophy) to deal with the overall well-being of the body directly through foods, herbs and meditation. I was given recipes to combine in my diet to boost my immune system and keep my body safe from the virus's attacks on my organs and respiratory system.

In addition, I practiced meditation which I have learned over the years and which I practice daily. My surprise was the spiritual journey I experienced, which went beyond my expectations, and which has had a lasting effect. I would have to admit, the breakthroughs of my soul's journey were a blessing as a result of this experience. It was in the quietness of the illness (from isolation and low oxygen) that profoundly enabled me to remove the sheath of illusion of this tangible "real" world scenario and face the intangible, my Creator. It came in the most creative manner with love, laughter, and beauty. I merged with the rain and floated on the feathers of birdsongs, while falling into a deep daydream. I found the way where beauty dwells in the Soul.

Recovery is harder than one can imagine and one should be aware that this virus lingers if not dealt with properly. As soon as I was ready for exercise and physical activity, I began the routine suggested by my medical doctor. It was slow, but steady. Then my heart began to bother me, so that's what I thought. I asked the doctor, a heart surgeon. She indicated it was normal to feel pressure on the heart due to the lung's lower capacity. I then asked for a specific routine from my yoga teacher for my heart and lungs. He alerted me to push the virus out of my lungs with a special aerobic yoga technique. I believe it is essential to treat the recovery period seriously, so as to overcome the virus fully without lasting effects or relapses. As I mentioned earlier, I began to show symptoms of the virus on Friday, March 13th.The following is an outline of my lessons learned.

39

Body

DURINGTHE VIRUS AND RECOVERY STAGES

My BODY:

* Studies mentioned in this section were researched post-recovery and are cited in the reference section.

Fever: The fever was a low-grade fever that never reached high temperatures, nor did I experience chills. It was annoying because it lasted longer (almost a week) than my usual fevers. In addition, it went almost undetected at first. Thus, I was moving around and not paying attention to its onset. I decided not to take aspirin nor inflammation reducers after the first day. I was alerted that it could create a worse condition, so I applied traditional remedies instead, mainly sleep, rest, and the determination to "grin and bear it". I kept tabs on my temperature to report to my doctor later. It was annoying as it lingered on, and on, and on. Patience is a virtue honed by experience. I had never had that kind of fever and in the past, I usually could take care of it with a couple of aspirins and go to work.

Recovery: Now I am careful not to overheat or catch cold that may trigger a fever. I stay out of the sun at noon and make sure I am dressed with a scarf for an early morning breeze. Also, I am more cautious about extreme changes in temperatures that may affect my body.

Kidneys: After the onset of the fever, my kidneys began to ache, and after the 3rd day the pain progressed to an unbearable suffering. I was curled up in a ball on the bed with excruciating sensations of a knife stabbing my lower back and going down my legs. It lasted for 5 days, along with the low-grade fever. My dehydration level was unbelievable! I kept two large thermoses by my bed with warm water (cold water was not recommended) and refilled them constantly. It never seemed like enough water, and yet surprisingly I was not eliminating the liquids! I had no chills and was not sweating. I was dumbfounded by this reaction. The ratio of water ingested to bathroom runs was completely "novel" and did not fit into my scheme of normalcy. Normally within an hour after drinking liquids I would be in the toilet. However, in this situation no bathroom runs were required. I lost track of my elimination process, but noted it was very low. Where the water was going, I have no idea!

A turmeric, black pepper and ginger drink from organic powders dissolved together in hot water was suggested by my yoga teacher, and I took it throughout the virus for my kidneys. At first, I tried this mixture early in the morning, but it was too harsh for my stomach. So, I changed to a midday option, as I used the mixture as a base for soups to save time and washing up duties. I just drank the mix (turmeric, black pepper, and ginger) first and then added water with garlic and other herbs like thyme or cumin. Finally, I cooked the vegetables for the soup. Chopped and boiled garlic recommended in Ayurveda released its antibacterial agents and worked well. Turmeric and ginger both supported my liver and kidneys for cells to face the challenge of the virus. This combination was also good for my lungs (anti- inflammation agents).

I found studies that supported this Ayurveda remedy with the following statements:

- "Turmeric, a spice that has long been recognized for its medicinal properties, has received interest from both the medical/scientific world and from culinary enthusiasts, as it is the major source of the polyphenol curcumin. It aids in the management of oxidative and inflammatory conditions, metabolic syndrome, arthritis, anxiety, and hyperlipidemia."
- "It may also help in the management of exercise-induced inflammation and muscle soreness, thus enhancing recovery and performance in active people. In addition, a relatively low dose of the complex can provide health benefits for people that do not have diagnosed health conditions. Most of these benefits can be attributed to its antioxidant and anti-inflammatory effects."
- "Ingesting curcumin by itself does not lead to the associated health benefits due to its poor bioavailability, which appears to be primarily due to poor absorption, rapid metabolism, and rapid elimination. But there are several components that can increase bioavailability. For example, piperine is the major active component of black pepper and, when combined in a complex with curcumin, has been shown to increase bioavailability by 2000%."

Recovery: I still go to bed with 2 large bottles of warm water at my bedside. One is filled with warm lemon water to drink upon waking up, and the other is filled with regular water or herbal tea. I drink warm lemon juice (made the night before and put by my bed in a thermos) at the start of the day in order to activate the bile from my liver. It takes time to change to alkaline, so that is why I drink it right away while

I'm still in bed. I began using some local herbal teas such as Dandelion and Horsetail (organic) to rejuvenate the liver and kidneys respectively. Now I continue using turmeric, ginger and black pepper to fortify my liver and kidneys. I pay close attention to my liquid intake, and I drink a minimum of 8 glasses a day on an empty stomach between meals, intermingled with herbal teas.

Lymph nodes: The overload on the lymph nodes of dead cells caused them to clog up. This resulted in my legs entering into a restless agony of shooting pains. I was awoken in the night due to pain running down each leg from all angles. I got up and danced, put them in the air, but to no avail. Finally, I remembered my yoga teacher explaining a lymph cleanse to apply to the skin. I made a homemade lymph scrub for my skin concocted from available spices in the kitchen such as mustard seeds, red rice, cinnamon, ginger, cumin. I rubbed it on my full body and dusted it off in the bathroom (messy. Then I applied soothing yogurt on my skin and followed this up with a warm shower. It did give me relief!

I began to pay attention to cleaning my skin more thoroughly (like a Japanese pre-bath scrub) to remove toxins. I did extra scrubbing in the shower as a daily routine no matter how dirty I felt. It was vital to keep up this routine in the morning after breakfast to rid my body of toxins accumulated on the skin. Lymph scrubs became a weekly ritual added to the virus challenge.

Recovery: I continue to scrub my skin well every shower. I take more showers to eliminate toxins on my skin, especially after waking up, after physical activity and before going to bed. I keep my spices stocked for lymph scrubs and yogurt for the finishing touch to soothe my skin.

Liver: Ironically, I had been aware of my liver through taking anti-malaria pills while working in a refugee camp in Thailand (sometimes quoted as a Covid-19 remedy). Unaware of the main ingredient and its long-term effect, it resulted in weakening my liver to the point of exhaustion and dizziness. It took me 14 years to recover. But luckily the liver is an organ that rejuvenates. I was able to understand when my liver was attacked by this virus mainly due to the sudden and extreme lack of energy I experienced. It felt like I was hit by 10 trucks. I added a dose of turmeric (fat soluble) to my yogurt knowing the powerful Ayurveda remedy would boost the liver vitality as a counter attack to the virus.

I found studies that explained the positive effects of turmeric on the liver in the following statements:

- "There are several plausible mechanisms that suggest the favourable effect of curcumin on liver function. Reports have indicated that oxidative stress and immune system disorder play important roles in contributing to liver dysfunction such as NAFLD.35 In this case, curcumin can improve oxidative stress and prevent NAFLD by decreasing production of reactive oxygen species, the hepatic protein expression of oxidative stress, pro-inflammatory cytokines, and chemokines such as interferon (IFN) γ, interleukin-1β and IFNγ-inducible protein 10.36, 37."
- "Cell-based studies have demonstrated the potential of turmeric as an antimicrobial, insecticidal, larvicidal, antimutagenic, radioprotector, and anti-cancer agent. Turmeric has also been used to support liver function and to treat jaundice in both Ayurvedic and Chinese herbal medicine."
- "Research during the past decade has identified numerous chemical entities from turmeric, and modern science has provided a logical basis for the safety and efficacy of turmeric against human diseases. Epidemiologic data indicate that some extremely common cancers in the Western world are much less prevalent in regions (Southeast Asia, e.g.) where turmeric is

> widely consumed in the diet. This spice has been found to be well tolerated at gram doses in humans. Dietary turmeric contains over 300 different components."

In addition, I ate as many bitter foods as possible during the process, such as locally grown artichokes and asparagus. Bitter foods are helpful to the liver, also.

***Recovery*:** My prior experience to rejuvenate my liver was drinking 1 litre of dandelion herbal tea over the course of the day, spread out from morning to late afternoon. In this case of the virus, it has been quite useful to apply the same remedy. I rotated two herbal teas for liver and kidney recovery (dandelion and horsetail) on alternate weeks. I imagine it will take 3 months for the liver and kidneys to fully recover. Hence, I have avoided coffee all through the virus and during this recovery period, as it puts too much pressure on these weakened organs.

Digestion: My past travels through Asia have been a double edge sword, with enhanced lessons of gastrointestinal challenges and ancient wisdom for the digestive tract. On one hand, I learned to starve out virus or bacteria induced digestive problems with plain white rice. Curiously enough, I had just bought some organic white rice (due to lack of brown rice) and readily had it available for the first few weeks of the virus. Then I noted the strange stench and coloration of my bowel movements, no comparison to other illnesses. In any case, I was too sick to really care. I had lost most of my smell and taste buds but oddly enough the smell was noticeably potent. I did not have diarrhoea actually, but loose enough to not be normal. I watched for changes and took notes on dietary complications. I began to notice oil and raw vegetables were problematic, so I eliminated them, even high-quality olive oil. I boiled or steamed my food. For oils, I only used organic butter on toast and added trail mix with nuts to my oatmeal breakfasts and midday snacks during activities (physical or mental work). I avoided salads or raw veggies, and cooked everything. This kept my spleen healthy by keeping watery foods to a minimum, and resulted in avoiding inflammation. I ate raw fruits at breakfast, mid-morning before yoga and bedtime (bananas).

It was vital to keep my body on the dry side, so these three rations of fruit throughout the day were enough to balance my diet for fibre and minerals. I remembered oatmeal was good for detox from a cancer chemotherapy recovery diet used by friends. I changed my meal portions not to overwhelm the digestive system and spread them out a bit to give time for digestion. Citrus fruits (lemon, orange, kiwi) were given 20 minutes to digest in order to make the transition from acid to alkaline to provide a strong immune system. (Never taken with dairy products, including vitamin C). I eliminated all dairy in order not to clog the lymph system, except one yogurt a day. I felt I needed the probiotics to rebuild the digestive process. I also harvested my own young green chilies and added them to my diet.

I found studies that supported Ayurveda green chilli remedy with the following statements:

- "People who eat chili peppers on a regular basis appear to lower their risk of dying from heart disease, a new study finds. Researchers analyzed the diets and health records of more than 22,000 people living in southern Italy and followed them for a median of just over eight years. People who ate chili peppers more than four times a week were about one-third less likely to die of heart disease than those who rarely or never ate the spicy-hot peppers. This protective benefit was evident regardless of whether people followed a Mediterranean-style diet (which is often recommended for heart health) or a less healthful diet. Chili peppers get their heat from a compound called capsaicin, which may help dampen inflammation and other harmful processes involved in the buildup of fatty plaque in arteries, according to the authors. Their study appeared Dec. 24, 2019, in the *Journal of the American College of Cardiology*." (Harvard University, March 2020).

- "When you bite into a pepper, the capsaicin attaches to a receptor that communicates with other cells. That communication causes a nerve on your tongue to immediately tell your brain that it's hot. That same receptor is found in your digestive tract. When capsaicin enters your digestive tract and attaches to the receptor, it creates a chemical called anandamide. Anandamide has been shown to lead to less inflammation in the gut, which can be caused by conditions such as ulcerative colitis and Crohn's disease. The same reaction that calms down your gastrointestinal tract may also keep it tumor-free. It may be particularly effective for people that are at high risk of developing intestinal tumors — such as people with a family or personal history of tumors." (University of Pennsylvania 2019).

Recovery: I continued the little to no dairy routine (a bit of milk with ginger tea and one yogurt). I waited 3 months to reintroduce salad into my diet. I began with a tiny bit of lettuce and cucumber (good to counter acidic foods). I continue with small portions. I continued to space out proteins and vegetables to give time for digestion for each food group. For example, after yoga I have a protein and then take a shower. That is time enough to allow the stomach to concentrate only on the digestion of the protein before overloading it with the next group of veggies. I try to thoroughly chew each food to give the stomach the signal from the saliva glands to release the appropriate enzyme to aide proper digestion. I began an appetizer yogurt lassi (no sugar or honey) that is just 4 parts water whipped with one-part yogurt to create the original "buttermilk" before lunch. The turmeric and black pepper drink was added with this appetizer to prepare my stomach for my main meal.

I began a cucumber, tomato, green pepper and green chilli drink (Gazpacho) after yoga on the hottest days of summer (July-August) to cool down as an appetizer. Young green chillies are good for the digestive tract (Ayurveda). I also began a 10-day probiotic regimen, other than the yogurt, to build up the flora in my stomach, which had deteriorated significantly.

Lungs: At one point (2 weeks) I began to realize that my lungs had a strange sensation. Clinically, it would be termed "shortness of breath". Poetically, I can only describe it as an open window in the lower half of my lungs. Perhaps this form of naming it from a poet's point of view was less dire. However, for me that was a turning point to drastically modify my activity because it did not get any better after a few days. In fact, it got worse. I believe it was a combination of denial and crisis management that I gave this symptom less attention. As part of the Covid-19 national health plan we had been given the ability to call a special telephone number to request medical attention at home or an ambulance to go to the hospital 24/7. Shortness of breath was the major reason to make that call. I suppose I was not ready to give up, so I attempted to use the old-fashioned rest-in-bed remedy. I was thrown back to the days of black and white cinema as a child when characters stayed in bed sleeping to fight off illness.

I stopped all activity that was not essential and only made use of the morning for breakfast, shower, meditation and lunch preparation. Each activity was slow and calculated. Day by day I noticed my inability to hold my breath in my daily yoga breathing exercises (pranayama). I laughed my way through these exercises and realized that the virus had hit my lungs. I stopped all physical yoga. I was in bed by 2-3pm. I sat in bed with pillows to prop me up in order to keep airways open. I began to read online literary magazines with poetry or short films that I never had time to enjoy. I found an old book given to me by my best friend on my bookshelf that I never had time to read. Tucked inside was a sweet note. It was almost the first book I found and it was perfect; A poetic style of short stories written last century with a slow rhythm by Kahlil Gibran, author of the *Prophet*.

I began to worry as the days lingered on. My doctor was concerned and in touch more often. Mentally I was hitting the wall. I reviewed my life wondering if I had really completed it sufficiently. Had I contributed enough to society? In addition, I was wondering if to alleviate my lungs, vapor steam over the stove with a towel was a good method or not? It turned out not to be a good remedy. No relief. I actually had no congestion or water. A friend suggested a simple remedy, which was to gargle with apple cider vinegar and swallow a bit, too. I did that and it seemed to help along with the rest. I was lucky to find organic apple cider vinegar in the local supermarket. There were many items understocked, but there was the vinegar I needed! I had picked up a bottle thinking it would be good to have on hand for the lockdown. (I also found fresh turmeric in the old market place, a rare item. I never saw it again after April). Amazing grace.

This phase easily lasted 2 weeks. I monitored my breath capacity with an attempt at a deep knee bend in the morning in the fresh air on my balcony. In my pranayama practice I took note of how much I could do before gasping for air. It seemed like forever before I could do a deep knee bend or get through 50% of my pranayama. I just had to be patient. I was so tired of being tired. Family, friends and yoga friends were constantly there on social media to boost my positive attitude, and they checked in several times a day, especially my friend from Italy. She seemed to know exactly what I was experiencing, as the pandemic was ravaging Northern Italy at the same time. I could not talk, too much energy. I never really got a cough per se. I just had a lot of dry throat clearing. I rejoiced the day I could do a deep knee bend on my balcony along with the sunrise. I began to salute the sun everyday with my new lungs! I remember the day I could dance! April 21st.

The semi-bed ridden phase to fight the virus in my lungs was devastating on my leg muscles. I had to relearn how to walk. My brain also was affected with swelling and yet I had a beautiful spiritual side effect in those moments of semi-consciousness.

Recovery: After 5 weeks I was so depleted from the virus having taken its course around my body, especially the last attack on my lungs. When it subsided, it was like stepping off a space ship back to Earth. I began to feel a desire to exercise. Questions arose about how much? My doctor sent me a recovery plan. Given the scare with the lungs, I was extra careful about exercise. I began with the slow arm and leg routines suggested by the physical therapy handout. The routines seemed pathetic for an athletic person like myself. However, I was aware of my limits and actually was in a self- care mode to treat myself delicately. Then I felt a pressure on my heart that was worrying. This is another Covid-19 symptom that sends people to the hospital. I consulted my doctor friend, a heart surgeon taking on follow- up Covid-19 patients, to ask about the situation. She assured me that it was normal given the lung's lower capacity. So, I was calmer.

Then I consulted my yoga teacher. I was in this super slow, careful mode of recovery. I wanted some sweet Hatha yoga (relaxing positions) for the heart. His suggestion floored me. He said, "Do fast yoga and breathe out loud through your mouth". I had to confirm his text message. He had been teaching us the "Fire breathing" technique for the past two years, called Bhastika. His Kundalini Tantra yoga is a combination of movement (mainly pelvic and shoulder regions) with breath release for emotional blockages in the body. I thought, I could barely walk, so now he wanted me to do "fast yoga"? He explained that the virus could be stuck between the heart and the lungs and it was vital to push it out to avoid lingering effects. He's never been wrong in 25 years, so I had a go at it.

I made my own routine of 12 minutes of aerobic yoga based on his techniques of hip and shoulder movements with exaggerated breathing to push out the virus. As a warm-up I used my bicycle to walk up the three flights of stairs to my apartment, or I walked up with my groceries to work up a sweat before doing this yoga. I ate fruit (kiwi) just before to give me an energy boost and waited 15 minutes for digestion. Then, I set my stopwatch and began this "novel" approach. It worked! I got stronger day by day.

Brain: My oxygen levels were significantly depleted due to my lower lung capacity, and my brain was less functional. I dozed off more easily in those afternoons and could not concentrate. In fact, I began to enter into a strange mode of consciousness. The material world began to matter less and less. Days of being in bed in the afternoons merged into a single moment.

Before I contracted the virus, I was working non-stop, commuting to Madrid from early morning and returning late at night most days. On weekends, I used to look at my bedroom with the lovely light shining through the lace curtains on the south window with a desire to take a nap. I hadn't extra time for such frivolity, back then. I had to catch up on housework, shopping, and preparing for the week with washing my clothes. Now, with this virus, it seemed like God's joke on me. I was taking extended naps every day! Covid-19 had converted my bedroom into a nursery room for long afternoon naps. (*Be careful what you wish for*).

With this virus, swelling of the brain, as much as I can ascertain, is normal for some patients. I had to lay with my head over the side of the bed to let blood rush into my brain for relief. I could not talk for more than 30 minutes. At the start of this virus attack, I had a massive headache during the fever phase. Then it changed into a general languid mental state during the lung phase. I could not work more than one hour online or do computer tasks. I limited all mental activity to a minimal.

I consulted my doctor, who assured me it was normal given my lower oxygen levels and the effects of my body being confined indoors. She encouraged me to be sure the house was well ventilated and to get outside for fresh air. She was confident it would improve with activity in the fresh air.

Recovery: On May 2nd we were able to do exercise outdoors! What a day to rejoice! I rode my bicycle along the tree-lined country roads with birds in the fields, enjoying the late Spring. (Thank goodness I had purchased a bike just before lockdown). Walking was very difficult on my legs due to muscle mass depletion whereas bike riding was easier. Riding a bike in the early morning was so wonderful for my brain and lungs! I still was very careful about overtaxing the brain. I continued to do the aerobic yoga exercises and fire breathing to increase lung capacity. I put my head over the side of the bed every night for a few minutes until my brain felt normal. In addition, I began to use the Ayurveda practice called the "neti pot" for cleansing my sinuses. It consists of a warm salt water wash of nose nostrils. It is recommended once a week by my yoga teacher to flush out the crystals that build up from toxins in the air. Pranayama daily practice clears the airways and facilitates this type of flushing of the nostrils more easily.

Then as I was recuperating, I rented a plot of land to farm that was physically and mentally enjoyable, and I began to get plenty of fresh air and sunshine. Nature was silently soothing to my mental state and farming kept me focused on a task with joy! It was an extension of my mini garden at home that I had started in lockdown. My yoga teacher is also a farmer in his spare time and says that Nature always gives you "love". It was perfect for healing my brain in a transition from the intangible dreamy state to the tangible realm.

I began this book as a way to get my brain back in the game, but in the slow lane. Poetry has been easy for me since I began to write as a child, so it was a wonderful way to recover. I did not worry about too many details. I just set up a simple plan of 3 poems for each chapter. I tried to make it pleasurable and helpful for people at the same time. It has been a magical experience to write this book from a virus that threw me into a whirlwind and my brain into a void. Strangely enough, it was the very disconnection of the brain that prompted a new path in my spiritual journey (*See Soul* section).

Bone marrow: After consulting various studies of Covid-19, I found some useful information about how the virus could have affected my bone marrow. Red and white blood cells are produced in the bone marrow along with platelets (blood clotting cells). When this system is under attack or overworked, it is inefficient or non-functioning. For example, in some cases, blood clots appear throughout the body's organs. Dead cells or abnormal ratio of immature cells accumulate in the lymph glands and spleen. I am not sure exactly what percentage of these complications I experienced, but the low energy (lack of red blood cells) and overloaded lymph nodes (dead cells) was apparent. I was aware of being on the lookout for heart changes as it was a deadly warning sign of complications from the virus (blood clots). I found that I needed to go to bed early to avoid depletion and generally my energy did not last past 7:00 pm. I got into a habit of going to bed super early. It meant I got up earlier, and with the birds singing outside my window it was a pleasure. It seemed to be a natural part of life.

The following statements are from the studies I encountered, and gave me an insight into bone marrow as a result:

- "Coronaviruses are able to infect bone marrow cells, resulting in abnormal hematopoiesis. Hematopoiesis: The production of all types of blood cells including formation, development, and differentiation of blood cells. Hematopoiesis is the production of all of the cellular components of blood and blood plasma. It occurs within the hematopoietic system, which includes organs and tissues such as the bone marrow, liver, and spleen. Simply, hematopoiesis is the process through which the body manufactures blood cells. In adults, hematopoiesis of red blood cells and platelets occurs primarily in the bone marrow. In infants and children, it may also continue in the spleen and liver."

- "A low white blood cell count usually is caused by viral infections that temporarily disrupt the work of bone marrow."
- "A low white blood cell count usually means your body isn't making enough white blood cells. It can increase your risk of all sorts of infections."
- "Bone marrow is the tissue comprising the centre of large bones. Damaged pulmonary capillary beds cause the process of megakaryocyte rupture and platelet release to be blocked, which affects the release of platelets into the pulmonary circulation and indirectly leads to reduced platelet synthesis in the systemic circulation."
- "Neutrophils are the first defense against invading microorganisms. Increased susceptibility to common pathogens has usually been attributed to extremely low counts (below 0.5×109/l) and individuals with "low normal" counts or ethnic neutropenia have not been reported to be at increased risk as long as counts are not further decreased. However, the probability to contract tuberculosis from patients with open pulmonary disease was inversely correlated with baseline neutrophil counts in a recent study."
- "Neutrophil counts in blood are determined by the differentiation and proliferation of precursor cells in the bone marrow, release of mature neutrophils into the blood, margination in organs like the lung and spleen, and transmigration through

the endothelial lining followed by neutrophil apoptosis and uptake by phagocytes. ”

- “The bone marrow is where new blood cells are produced. Bone marrow contains two types of stem cells: hemopoietic (which can produce blood cells) and stromal (which can produce fat, cartilage and bone). There are two types of bone marrow: red marrow (also known as myeloid tissue) and yellow marrow. Red blood cells, platelets and most white blood cells arise in red marrow; some white blood cells develop in yellow marrow. The colour of yellow marrow is due to the much higher number of fat cells.”
- “In cases of severe blood loss, the body can convert yellow marrow back to red marrow in order to increase blood cell production. Lack of red blood cells causes the body to draw from yellow marrow to convert back to red marrow to produce red blood cells (oxygen carriers). Yellow marrow is designed to produce fat and tissue after the age of five. Fat and muscle mass reduction result from inactivity (bed ridden-muscle mass loss) and lack of production from yellow marrow (fat cells) in order to help red blood marrow, produce healthy red cells.”
- “Red blood cells, white blood cells, and platelets are all produced in the red bone marrow. As we age, the distribution of red and yellow bone marrow changes. Bone marrow’s highest production in adults is located in the shoulder, pelvic and spine areas of the human body bone structure.”
- “After production of white blood cells in bone marrow, these cells need to move freely to fight off infection. These cells circulate better throughout the body with the head down, and the trunk inverted through specific yoga positions. For example, a “downward dog” position is recommended by yoga experts.”
- “Our bodies don't make vitamin C, but we need it for immune function, bone structure, iron absorption, and healthy skin.

We get vitamin C from our diet, usually in citrus fruits, strawberries, green vegetables, and tomatoes."

- "Sleep plays a major role in repair work on the human body. There's a substantial body of evidence that stress weakens the immune system and makes us vulnerable to infection and disease, so there is a relationship between sleep and a healthy immune system, and the damage that a lack of sleep can have. While more sleep won't necessarily prevent you from getting sick, skimping on it could adversely affect your immune system, as the immune system kicks into action during that time. The natural rhythm for reparation is 10-11pm."

Recovery: Turmeric and ginger are full of iron, which is needed to produce red and white blood cells. In turn these cells support the immune system as well as rejuvenate the organs, including muscle rebuilding. The yoga program that I followed is based on breathing and movement. I remain vigilant on sleep patterns for maximum health.

My yoga teacher combines Ayurveda (diet) and asanas (body positions) to lead a healthy life. He created his own version of yoga called kundalini tantra yoga (*see reference section*) that is focused on movement (original tantra yoga) and breathing (kundalini+prananyama). His routines focus especially on the tailbone and hips (pelvic region) and shoulders, to build red blood cells. In fact, he uses a rolling motion of the shoulders and circular pelvic movements in many positions. Only after studying about bone marrow was I aware of the science of his yoga. He is constantly telling us that "life is in the tailbone."

My yoga teacher has modified the "downward dog" yoga position by emphasising movement to avoid stagnant blood build up in the brain combined with more spinal movement, and tailbone action. His form of downward dog position is practiced with swinging movements. This helps to activate the shoulders, spine and tailbone at the same time.

I used Echinacea as an immune booster in recovery in a tincture form. This has been a powerful preventative tool in my past in times of stress. However, it seemed relevant in recovery given the depletion of my immune system. I started in May, and will end in August (two months only).

Foods high in Vitamin C were especially important to me on a daily basis. I ate an orange in the morning (waited 20 minutes to digest it and transform it to alkaline), drank warm lemon juice upon waking, and before my yoga workout I ate 1-2 kiwis. I also took a Vitamin C supplement during the peak of the virus for 2 months. Lemon grass tea or papaya were recommended by my yoga teacher but I was not able to obtain these items. Now tomatoes will soon be in season, along with green peppers. These foods will naturally boost my immune system as they will be infused with the rich sunshine from the full summer growing season, fresh from my garden!

I go to bed early enough to be sleeping by 10pm. If fatigued, I get into bed earlier to compensate for winding down time, 1.5 hours before. If not fatigued mentally, I can slip into a slumber sleep easily within 30-45 minutes. I wake up early and attend to my garden, a farmer's timetable, in harmony with the sun's natural rhythm. I actually wake up before sunrise for optimal energy, and capitalize on the sun's energy propelling me into the day. I prefer this tactic to running behind the sun, late rising.

Muscle mass: My fever was very low but my muscles ached more than past experiences I have had with a normal fever and chills. I had never had chills or sweats at night. I was dehydrated from the whole virus process. My body mass dropped 9 kilos (20 pounds) in 3 weeks, even though I ate carbs and sat around with having done little exercise. I was amazed at the fat and muscle loss my body experienced! I could barely walk, and felt like I had to re-learn walking due to the loss of leg muscles. My first days out to go shopping, I remember having trouble taking a slow stroll just 2 blocks away to the grocery store. Climbing the 3 flights of stairs with shopping bags to my apartment was arduous.

I dreaded going out for anything, but I had run out of fresh food. It took me so long to get dressed! I could not stand up for more than 5 minutes. Also, it was also agony cooking on my feet and I had to sit down several times during these ordinary tasks, not to mention my brain functioning in slow motion. I had to prepare my bag, gloves, mask, coat, shoes and shopping cart. Upon returning, I had to strip down clothes and shoes in the entrance hall, unload my shopping cart, wipe down all the items, and then disinfect the shopping cart and my shoes.

Note: To be socially responsible I quarantined 2 weeks after the fever subsided. A friend from Madrid kindly came to my rescue with bags of groceries, when I ran out of fresh fruits and vegetables after 10 days. (Our lockdown was scheduled for 10 days, so I only bought enough for that period). In hindsight I would have cooked food and frozen it. For fresh fruits, I would have cut up and frozen them, or made smoothies to freeze in zip-lock bags. It was seemed vital for my body to have these foods to replenish my muscles. Looking then at the empty refrigerator was not a pleasant experience. I have usually fended for myself, but I had to admit I was out of time and fresh food. Later I found out the local network of shoppers and shops that delivered. The large grocery shops delivered but did not have online shopping. It was complicated. I was new in the town and could not go out to ask neighbours. I was astounded by the loss of body mass in such a short time and the importance of exercise for my immune system.

I read some studies on the subject and found the following:

- "During an infection, the body becomes catabolic (the opposite of anabolic) and breaks down muscle protein. The degree of muscle catabolism and protein loss is related to the height and duration of the fever caused by the infection."

- "The amino acids that are liberated from the muscles are scavenged by the liver and used as an emergency energy source (glucose production via gluconeogenesis) and as the building blocks for acute phase proteins, which the body employs to fight infection."
- "Your muscles have many good reasons to ache when you have an infection. Skeletal muscle is the main source of catabolized protein, but heart muscle contributes as well."
- "Studies have shown a 25 percent decrease in isometric muscle strength after a simple febrile illness such as the flu. Replenishing muscle mass lost during a three-day febrile illness may take up to two weeks."
- "According to the adjustment of the exercise protocol, it can cause temporary microtraumas of varying degrees in skeletal muscles [5, 6]. These skeletal muscle microtraumas induce the tissue regeneration process. In this process, immune cells such as neutrophils and macrophages are activated to work in the recovery of tissue homeostasis, producing pro- and anti-inflammatory mediators."
- "Over the past two decades, a variety of studies has demonstrated that exercise induces considerable physiological change in the immune system. Acute and chronic exercise alters the number and function of circulating cells of the innate immune system (e.g., neutrophils, monocytes, and natural killer (NK) cells)."
- "There is a straight relationship between exercise and the immune system. Exercise may modulate the immune system response acutely and chronically. Nevertheless, physical exercise also induces the release of myokines in the blood circulation. The physiological function of myokines produced by the skeletal muscle is to protect and improve the functionality of many organs. Furthermore, there is convincing evidence that factors

secreted by the skeletal muscle act as endocrine signalling mediators and are involved in the beneficial effects of exercise on almost all cell types and organs."

- "Cellular response is immediate after exercise. A significant increase in total leukocyte, neutrophil, monocyte and lymphocyte counts was observed immediately following all three types of exercise. Prolonged exercise induced the greatest increase in total circulating leukocyte, neutrophil and monocyte counts, but peak aerobic exercise induced a similar increase in lymphocyte counts; lesser responses in all cell subsets were provoked by resistance exercise."
- "As a powerful extensor of the hip joint, the gluteus maximus suited to powerful lower limb movements such as stepping onto a step, climbing or running but is not used greatly during normal walking. Gluteus maximus and the hamstrings work together to extend the trunk from a flexed position by pulling the pelvis backwards, for example standing up from a bent forward position. Eccentric control is also provided when bending forward. Superior fibres of the gluteus maximus can extend the knee through its attachment to the Iliotibial tract."'
- "Gluteus maximus has several stability roles: balancing the pelvis on femoral heads thus maintaining upright posture, the attachment through the iliotibial tract supports the lateral knee, and lateral rotation of femur when standing assists raising the medial longitudinal arch of the foot."

Recovery: Production of muscle mass to replace loss from deterioration (a virus side effect) was essential for my body. After May 2nd when the lockdown was lifted and outdoor exercise was allowed, excursions were part of my early morning daily routine, mainly with my new bicycle. The fresh air was heavenly! My bike was a godsend, as I could not manage a walk for cardio exercise. It was too hard for long distances and I did not feel my lungs or muscles benefited from short walks, nor my mind. The only drawback from the bike ride was the hefty lifting of the bicycle on my shoulder up the 3 flights of stairs to my apartment! This took some practice and every day I felt stronger. I used this strength test as a gauge of my progress in building muscle mass.

Yoga workouts for cardio was the first thing I did after a bike ride or shopping excursion. I was warmed up, especially after climbing up the stairs to my apartment with my bicycle or shopping cart full of groceries (kilos of fruits and veggies). After the cardio workout, I did yoga positions for muscle toning and ligaments. Then I finished with the "fire breathing" pranayama and specific yoga for organ rejuvenation (kidney, liver, spleen) and digestive track. I followed my yoga teacher's program in Kundalini Tantra yoga. At first, I could only do 30 minutes divided equally between cardio (12 min) and fire breathing (8 min), toning (7 min). Note: It was important to do the cardio and muscle toning prior to pranayama breathing because releasing the toxins (pranayama) is best after the blood is warmed up/flowing and joints are lubricated.

After 6 weeks of exercise, in mid-July, I could walk 10 kilometres (6 miles) without fatigue. I felt my legs had recovered and my lungs as well. Now I often take a stroll in the afternoon after lunch, and continue the early, morning bike ride to the organic farm, rejoicing in the fresh air. I weighed close to 59 kilos (132 lbs.) at the start and now in mid-July, 51(113 lbs). I actually feel younger and more vibrant with my new body mass! My yoga has improved tremendously due to my lighter body, especially with the loss of the largest muscle mass, gluteus maximus.

40

Mind

My mindset in this ordeal was key to the outcome of making decisions and controlling how to approach each situation that arose. My body was in pain and under strain from having to battle with rapidly changing symptoms. A "novel" virus meant it took over my being, running a course unknown to both my mind and my body. I had years of practice with colds, coughs, flu, upset stomachs, muscle pain and many other conditions I have had to deal with in the past. Nevertheless, this virus ran a sequence that was totally bizarre to me. I could not predict how to prepare for each new phase. In fact, it was impossible to confront it with experiences from the past and without a pattern. The fear factor was definitely part of Covid-19 that is present in some moments more than others. Even if you go to the hospital, how can they help you? Other than emergency care, with no antibiotics or cure, I had to just face each phase as it hit my body. However, I am convinced that my mindset from the beginning was a blessing thanks to my yoga teacher and friends. I believe that the three most important elements of my mentality were 1) Laughter, 2) Inspiration and 3) Mindfulness.

Laughter

I had already lost job contracts due to Covid-19 earlier in the week before I had my first symptom, the fever. It had put me into a downward motion of negativity and emotional havoc of worry. That lasted 2 days before I pulled myself out of that hole and started to think differently. Now I had more time and the weather was gorgeous. This was before lockdown. I bought a bike, and started to ride around the countryside. I had more time to dedicate to yoga and get my house in order after an arduous winter schedule of commuting to Madrid. I was feeling quite positive going into the lockdown. In addition, I had just watched a short video clip of my yoga teacher talking about Covid-19 with a smile and laughing. He was proposing that our bodies are like a container to process the negative, so we should just let it go through its course. He viewed it as a learning process of how much you can process negative energy without being affected. He also remarked, "Be Smart". He was laughing, in fact about it, to help us be less afraid. It worked for me.

In the first few days of my fever and pain in the legs I was keeping up with a jovial attitude in order to process the negative and just let it flow through me. Indeed, it was painful and uncomfortable, but my yoga teacher's face and smile stuck with me. Actually, I did not tell a lot of people what I was going through. I did not want to a victim. My landlord jokingly said that his sister "probably had it, and we all would eventually get it." He was also light about it. It turned out his sister did have it and her two-year-old daughter, but they went through it mildly. Anyway, both my landlord and my yoga teacher from the onset were my lighthouses to keep light about it. I mimicked them and began to focus on laughter.

I had remembered a cancer doctor who recommended funny videos or books to help the brain stay uplifted during chemotherapy and all the process of the disease. It really matters how the brain reacts to situations to create a chemical chain of reactions in the body. Laughing produces endorphins that boost the immune system, or at least does not deplete it.

I began to ask friends to send me only jokes on social media and leave out the political or depressing news of the virus. There were plenty of political controversies roaming around the world wide web entangling people into debate. I wanted to stay away from that type of burden on my brain. Most people were kind and stopped sending messages of that sort. I had a few friends who really understood and sent me at least one joke a day, or more. I cherished these messages. I re-sent them to others and we were all laughing. I even translated for others to enjoy. The Spanish people are very clever and witty, with Don Quixote as a benchmark. Homemade videos and images were hilarious. I was alone in my quarantine but laughing aloud! I got a good daily dose a few times a day. I feel this attitude was essential in keeping my body reacting favorably to each phase.

Inspiration

Inspiration comes in many packages. In leadership training it's called motivation. In healing it's called affirmations. In sports it's called "do another lap" and then shoot the free throw (when you're tired). I have been exposed to all these types of inspiration, and more. In yoga it's a little different. It's called Bhakti yoga. You offer yourself and this inspires others to do the same. It is modelled from the moon, as the moon only reflects the light of the sun, offering a vessel for a light in the dark. A lighthouse has the same function. This type of inspiration is the first step towards helping others and then it creates a ripple effect. Eventually it comes back as love from the universe.

I began to send inspirational social media texts in the mornings and evenings. I was going to bed early and waking up early with the birds, so I started with this image. I looked for beautiful birds as a symbol of springtime. I sent out a message of "Good Morning, Buenos Dias". In the evening I looked for calming images of sunsets with "Good night, Buenos Noches." It was also a way to keep tabs on everyone I cared about. I created my "tribe" individually and not a WhatsApp group. I wanted people to have their privacy respected. It took a bit of finger tapping, but it was worth it!

During the pandemic people seemed to be bored, anxious, and worried about gaining weight. I sent them funny dance videos, recipes, or other music to inspire them to be positive. They responded and we were tapping away our worries. I truly appreciated all those messages and the effort people took to keep my spirit high. They also made sure I was okay. I am sure they were worried. There seemed to be endless beautiful birds with flowers in springtime to send every day. I even recorded the birdsongs outside my window! I did change to lotus flowers, butterflies, horses and other nature images. I found some classical music to be very inspiring, such as Handel. All in all, I was so grateful for my "tribe "and the mutual inspiration we shared. It is the end of July and I am still sending "Good Morning" almost every day.

Mindfulness

The original mindfulness is said to be a Buddhist concept. Buddha, having been a yogi striving for the best way to reach the end of suffering, discovered "the *middle way*". The middle way means not to be extreme, and is focused on the PRESENT, not past nor future. The mindfulness concept of being in the "now" is a reaction to the anxiety we face in a modern lifestyle that requires several skills to mitigate the fast pace presented on a daily basis, especially in urban settings.

In the past, a hyperactive person was considered abnormal. Today this "normal" behavior is called "multi-tasking" and a dexterity that is rewarded! The hyper- lifestyle is exasperated by a global market that pushes the limits of our human capacity to keep up with the latest trends or productivity. We ourselves, myself included, overschedule and pack our timetables with little rest or space to even concentrate on the present task before moving on to the next objective (whether mentally or physically).

In the Covid-19 scenario, I was forced to utilize mindfulness due to my lack of energy and my limited brain function. It was highly useful to remember how to slow the mind down, a skill I had learned this in meditation. I was taught by my yoga teacher to not worry about the rambling mind, but to let it go. He recommended a split screen concept. In other words, try not to use the mind to calm the mind (almost impossible). He focused on the heart. You listen to your heart and focus on its connection to the universe. As the heart focus rises, the mind diminishes. I just had to keep my mind confined to avoid distractions.

I noticed that the mind is always reacting to the exterior impulses or visual cues that pulled it off task. I had to resist my mind that looked at a dirty corner of the house and wanted to clean it. I had to reel in its urges to do a load of wash after cleaning the bathroom. It was a time to slow, slow, slow down. I had to make schedules to keep myself healthy. Today I am washing clothes, which meant just flipping the switch and waiting to unload and hang dry. Tomorrow I am mopping the floors or dusting them. The next day I am cleaning the bathroom (essential only) and no deep cleaning. I kept my mind at bay from piling up tasks in one day. I spread out the housework.

Cooking was also a game changer in mindfulness. I had to create a couple of simple recipes for breakfast and lunch. After lunch I did not have any more energy. I opted for a fruit plate, peeling a banana and cutting up another fruit. That saved time washing dishes after dinner. Breakfast was slow and not rushed. I eliminated coffee and that helped me to be less anxious. Considering I had nothing to do and nowhere to go, coffee seemed overrated. Chopping vegetables took a lot of concentration so as to avoid cutting my fingers. So, I just did everything slowly and evenly. I was not sure how well my system could handle a cut or infection. Pots and pans were kept to a minimal, also. I used one plate, one bowl, one spoon, one fork and two knives. I did not leave any dishes overnight and less dishes meant easy to wash up.

I felt as if I was living in a long meditation. The house was silent, the apartment complex was silent, the streets were silent. However, that did not guarantee that my mind would be silent. I had to be vigilant and watch out for detours. I played some soft classical music to inspire me at times. I sang mantras lightly to keep my mind distracted to connect to the universe. I was lucky that I had already had some meditation skills. Nonetheless, the virus tested me. I had to apply all my knowledge from several channels to overcome a mental breakdown, especially living through the virus alone in isolation.

41

Soul

"Yesterday we complained about Time and trembled. But today we have learned to love it and revere it, for we now understand its intents, its natural disposition, its secrets, and its mysteries. Yesterday we were a toy in the hands of Destiny. But today Destiny has awakened from her intoxication to play and laugh and walk with us. We do not follow her but she follows us."

Kahlil Gibran (Thoughts and Meditations)

Silence-Awakening

Silence permeated the lockdown, mainly from shock. The numbers of cases and deaths rose like a tidal wave in Spain. Streets, apartment buildings, sidewalks, and all forms of the ordinary, jovial life of this country had ceased to exist in early Spring of 2020. March and April seemed like a long dragged out overture to an unfinished symphony Beethoven had heard tangled in his mind, but was afraid to commit to paper lest it be played out on a stage for all to hear. In the midst of this suspended time-frame, I swung in and out of reality. It was like parallel worlds, mine compared to that of my closest friends and family. Some were bored, anxious, and confused by the first weekend (5 days into lockdown). Others felt that the Coronavirus was a mystery blowing in the wind out there on the horizon, but surreal from their line of view.

I was beyond their time and space. I was in a bubble shared by 66,000 other cases in Madrid. We were silent partners at an epicentre in this pandemic. Quite early on, I lost my energy to speak, so I was immersed in silence in an ordinary home setting. As my energy dwindled, my steps were fewer and fewer, lighter and lighter. Thoughts were single layered, converging into an unspoken reality. It created a unique space, like in the lull after the music stops; a noiseless terrain. I cannot say it was a silent retreat because I had entered into this state without preparation. It was what it was; a silent film with an unfinished storyline.

As the days tallied up, I was washed away on a boat with no captain, no oars, no sails, and only the vast sea lit by a sliver of moonlight fading in and out as the waves carried me further and further out to an unknown horizon. I could only lie down in the bow of the boat and listen to heartbeats of mermaids imagined or real. Given that my heart rate was slowing down and my mind was unable to race around at its normal rate, I had no choice but to succumb to an altered subsistence. My brain activity was minimal, only working to do chores, routines, and heading to bed to rest. I did not even have the energy to be bored. Without trying anything, I was lying in my little boat (bed) and gracefully dropped into a hidden stratum of (un)reality. One rainy afternoon, I was overcome with a greater sensitivity for Beauty.

I was searching for inspiring images to send out for friends to say "Good Afternoon" when I found a blue lotus veiled in transparent petals that summed up my new inclination towards LIFE. I listened and watched the rain drops roll down my window outside and I merged with their essence as if the sheath between me and Nature had been magically removed. We were ONE. My heartbeat was mimicking those droplets, I was a silent witness to their destiny. I was AWAKE!

Heart Opening

"And I will give them one heart, and a new spirit I will put within them. I will remove the heart of stone from their flesh and give them a heart of flesh...

Genesis; Ezekiel 11:19

The heart of our planet is under the sea, where on the surface there are waves and sea spume crashing upon the shore. I have fond memories of floating and drifting in turquoise hues submerged in a tropical garland of sea friends, while swimming in one of the seven seas on the equator. I have been touched by sea grass brushing lightly across my arm and astounded by the essence of Time; how it loosens underwater. It is a fleeting moment almost forgotten upon reaching the sounds of rippling waves behind me as I step onto the sand. It was a glimpse of what lies inside of my heart, hidden from even me, myself and I. The sea has always been the sense of true beauty to me. In the same way, my first experience with snowflakes was in Japan, where they were falling on a lotus pond. I was awakened by their nimble ballet outside my window. This surprising and exquisite phenomenon propelled my heart to move my body out of bed and witness the undisputable beauty just beyond my fingertips. It was an ephemeral moment, and yet has stayed with me over three decades. These are memories gathered in life that have given me sensory experiences with the heart of this planet in her beauty. (*See reference section for color pyshcology of turquoise*).

What does it mean to actually open your heart and merge with the heart of the planet and even the universe? In my meditations, this sense of union with the Cosmos has come and gone like fleeting experiences, only to end with the time allotted. Instinctively, I would close up the layers of bliss uncovered in meditation like closing up an onion, and then return to my ordinary, sometimes mundane life. It was a protective reaction to remain less vulnerable, I suppose. However, my experience with Covid-19 enabled my actual heartbeat and brain to slow down enough for an extended amount of time (days) opening me up to merge with the rain, the birdsongs and plant life in my mini-garden. It allowed me to pass over to a new perspective. I was still engrossed in the mundane tasks (who else was going to cook or clean?) and yet I carried this overwhelming sense of BEAUTY everywhere with me. On one hand I was facing death and on the other hand I was gently guided to a path of Beauty beyond my comprehension.

How did the stone heart crack, you ask? Under pressure from this virus, I say. I suppose how a diamond, in the deep isolated stratums of the Earth, is formed under pressure. Once the virus hit my lungs and possibilities of complications arose in my mind, I had to surrender or panic. I had reached a point of no return. It was a fork in the road. I called out in the middle of a stormy night for help from my Creator. Astounding me, the answer came almost immediately in the form of a loud crack, thunder! A lightning bolt lit up the sky. Then, I knew my

Creator was near, greater than the virus, and it was protecting me. I'll never forget that sound; and just at the right TIME.

Now in late July, I am still carrying this sense of BEAUTY with me. Finally, after years of practice in meditation, the clouds in my heart have vanished. I am no longer confused with a dual lifestyle, one in meditation and one in the mundane. The mundane is now a long meditation with a routine of tasks to make life easier. I would hope no one would have to wait as long as I.

However, it does seem to coincide with other literature that describe the necessity of experiencing extreme circumstances to reach Cosmic Bliss. It is usually described as a long process, but in the case of the virus we have been lucky; Covid-19 is here to speed that process along! I see it that way, with a smile. The fork in the road is behind me, and hopefully I will not find a detour to take me back to that unconscious place I lived in before. I prefer to continue bathing in the BEAUTY of the intersection where the inner (finite me) and outer (infinite Cosmic) heart commune. Six weeks of Covid-19 and 2 months of recovery have given me a chance for my stone heart to be weathered down, as the gates of stone around it crumble. The resulting rubble is the source for my cobblestone road that I am building as my path out of Covid-19. I wouldn't call it mundane struggling to fit all those stones together to make a solid road in a new direction. I call it "HEART BREAKING", and from here my heart is open to fuse with others, and share the road.

"Perhaps I need not part from the delightful world about me; when my body unites with the earth, my spirit may merge with this beauty. Mother Earth, I can see you going into your splendid chamber carrying me in your pure arms with maternal care and affection. I will lie in that arbour, listening to the mountain stream's song of peace. The trees and shrubs nearby will shower their blossoms on me." (Sita bids farewell to Rama).

Ramayana, Indian Epic

Healing my body from the inside out seemed dauntless in the midst of my isolation, with few options for caretakers, in fact none. Given my limited circumstance, I found solace in the tiniest contact with a living organism. I was waiting for my daffodil bulbs to bloom, staring at a large pot of soil, inactive. I had planted late, so blossoms would be in late April rather than February or March. I had not finished my back-porch project for plants and was caught off guard with a bit of leftover potting soil and two empty pots. I had been reading about growing plants, mainly sunflowers, like a far-off dream. Somehow, I found an article about growing plants from kitchen scraps like carrots and radishes. It was worth a try. I scrounged up enough soil for one pot and filled the second one halfway. I cut off the tops of a carrot and a radish to plant. I threw some mustard seeds in for fun to grow sprouts in one pot. I collected and dried some green pepper seeds from my cutting board and planted a few in the other pot. That was the only life I had to contemplate, and the potential plants became my new little friends. I greeted them in the morning checking on their progress and began to depend on them for a "real social life" beyond my virtual social thread with family and friends.

As they grew and struggled to reach the sunlight, I went through my Covid-19 rollercoaster. I began to greet them in the mornings to check on their progress and conversed with them as my companions. The radish was sprouting upward and branching out with new broad leaves. By its side the carrot was hanging in there to keep the radish company with its elegant, fanlike greenery. They were a cute couple. Meanwhile, the green peppers were burgeoning! The mighty mustard seeds were the fastest of them all, proliferating in both pots. My mini - organic garden was being born! My yoga teacher had told me if I wanted to start a farm, I should just begin with four posts and not worry at all. Strangely, I was starting my garden with four plants on a window sill.

My first harvest was filled with mixed emotions for me. After all I had created a friendship with these plants! They sustained me in the mornings and throughout the day. I could have sworn that they secretly assured me "everything was going to be alright." The blur of imagination and lack of social contact with real people made life surreal. Besides my world was already in slow motion with my lungs pumping less oxygen. Still, it was a wonderful relationship to cultivate on the south window, where beams of sunlight poured through to brighten my silence. Together these natural elements contributed to my sense of healing. I watched the bold effort of the plants breaking through the soil to find the light. My observations became more focused as the days merged together, and I realized that I could learn from their courage. There they were alone on a tiny spot of Earth dedicated to their mission; adapting to their circumstances. Needless to say, I began to clip some sprouts and radish leaves for an organic gourmet (meniscal) salad.

The radish and mustard sprouts kept producing as the green peppers brazenly reached out of the dark pot to the light. Poor things, they had a long way to go with only a half full container. The daffodils were shooting up alongside as the centrepiece. As the radish outgrew its purpose to produce a root bulb, it began to shoot up with flowering antennae. I was fascinated at its evolutionary changes over time. The wild configuration of these delicate branches was so remarkable. I witnessed this elaborated architectural design with balanced prongs moving in synchronicity outward in the four sacred directions. It was a primordial effort how the plants formulated a plan to cast their seeds. The final design was a horizontal pinwheel. I got so much pleasure out of this process. It transformed me from observer to team player with nature. I encouraged their growth and made sure they had water and sunlight, and when the green peppers were roasting in the south sun and wilting, I moved them to the north side where there was a breeze in the afternoons and more insect activity for pollination. I moved them back at night to be close to their friends to sleep. We spent a lot of quality time together, and it was a privilege to be amongst these earthlings.

I will never forget the day my first daffodil blossomed. She surprised me as a gift from the universe. It was just after my first bike ride, May 2nd. I was pumped up from the freedom ride in the early brisk morning air. As I was arriving home there on my porch was a beautiful bloom greeting me! I had not ever grown daffodils, so it was a "novel" experience. It was lovely to soak up its intricate design. In fact, its beauty baffled me!

I had not been very familiar with a daffodil up close. Sadly, I had shied away from Wordsworth's poem about the daffodils in my PhD study, thinking it was too cliché. I bypassed his poem for something more challenging. I ended up on the harrowing ledges of Hellvelyn, climbing up Swirral Edge and scuffling down by way of Striding Edge. What a contrast in life! Covid-19 had opened up my world to the subtle beauty of daffodils. Well, destiny is *a long and winding road*. Someday I would like to go back to the Lake District and see the ancestors of my daffodils from the bottom of the "watch towers" of Hellvelyn in the valley. Now, I feel I am ready and willing to surrender to the simple pleasures that nature has to offer.

My newfound relationship with nature during that slow-motion quarantine has stayed with me beyond lockdown. I was able to rent a plot of land (30x30 meters) and start an organic garden, encouraged by my new green friends. It became a wonderful way to recover my strength through sunshine and physical activity with a mission: eat by the labour of my own hands! I watched the butterflies appear from the wild fields next to my plot. They seemed so light and full of elegance fleeting from flower to flower. They had emerged from their cocoon as I from my quarantine. We both had wings and were lured to the nectar of flowers.

So now I began to plant my dreamy sunflowers. Some of the other gardeners planted a few to attract pollinators. I, however, planted a mini forest of sunflowers on either side to flank my plot. It is great joy to sit solidly on the Earth and feel fully embraced by her healing powers. I meditate every day in my garden, and say "thank you" and "I'm sorry." I do hope Mother Nature forgives me for not appreciating her gift of exquisite beauty wrapped up in a dormant bulb at the bottom of a patch of Earth. Her daffodil has been forever the inspiration for poets, and now for even a simpleton like me.

Grateful

We do not walk alone. Great Beings walk beside us. Know this and be Grateful.

-Polingaysi Qoyawayma, Hopi

May the stars carry your sadness away, may the flowers fill your heart with beauty, may hope forever wipe away your tears, And, above all, may silence make you strong.

– Chief Dan George, Tsleil-Waututh

I grew up with a boy who spent summers in the circle of Hopi elders, and this was my first introduction to indigenous wisdom; These memories have remained in the layers of my skin beyond primary school. My own mother was so enamoured with Native American (First Nations) art and culture. It became part of my belief system to honour the Earth with the Great Spirit in mind. "The truly wise know God by many names," says my yoga teacher. I am indebted for the array of spiritualities that have crossed my path, fostering my growth as a person. The experience with Covid-19, however brought out these values like a string of pearls dropped in the sea. Each one returning to its origin, leading me back to the fundamental values of LIFE. The sum of these philosophies is greater than one alone. Nonetheless, being thankful is a piercing sound amongst them all.

Honour your father, your mother, your elders, your teachers, Great Mother of the Earth, Great Spirit in the sky.

I would like to add to the list: Honour your friends.

The art of friendship is among one of the values of life that makes me grateful. Sharing experiences with friends over the years creates very special bonds. During this illness, I was reminded of how important these voices (or rather voiceless texts) cheered me up in order to battle Covid-19. There were a variety of friends sending me good thoughts and vibrations. Jokes were bouncing off the walls as we shared them, one after another. One friend caught me off guard on a depressing moment, and cheered me up to remember all my progress and not give up! It was a turning point. I will never forget that cheerleader!

I became aware of how foods and their amazing healing powers were gifts from Mother nature brought home to my kitchen. I used the wisdom of our elders who passed on the ancient recipes to immediately fight the enemy germs, and I could fight this virus effectively on time. It was a precise timing that boosted my red and white blood cells to do their tasks. I was faintly aware that a greater force than myself was at work deep inside my body.

I could not have kept a cool head without the sense of confidence my doctor friend gave me. She was in the eye of the Covid storm at a major hospital in Madrid. It was her advice and assurance that made it easier to keep plugging along, in a positive way. She would encourage me with small text messages, even though she was extremely busy. Actually, she was a heart surgeon who had to take on the responsibility of follow-up calls to Covid patients. In my case she only seemed to get worried when the virus hit my lungs. I had not been too worried, but her added questions were noted. I took them seriously and adapted my routine to rest more in the afternoons. She kept a low profile, but a steady one, and I did not bother her daily. Once in a while, I contacted her to confirm my symptoms and follow the right protocol. Since she had her pulse on the latest news of the epidemic, it was tremendously helpful to know I was within the norm. It was just a matter of riding out the wave. Some of her colleagues with the Covid symptoms had already been admitted to the hospital earlier and she was familiar with the course of the virus. I am ever appreciative for her cool, calm demeanour.

Women's motherly instincts seemed to have abounded during this process, as I had daily check-ins from important women in my life. I believe it was just natural. My older sister has always been like a second mother, and she listened to my endless texts when I was nervous. I think this was quite helpful to know someone was out there on the other side, a life line so to speak, without edits. I hope it did not bore her too much. I know she was worried, but she kept calm throughout the critical weeks. Other friends who are mothers took special moments to make sure I was responding to texts. They were especially attentive. My dear friend in nearby Italy was always nudging me if I did not send a text by 9 am. I know she was very worried as well. I am truly grateful for this seemingly added minor attention, but actually these contacts were great stepping stones to churning milk into butter so I could climb out of my hole.

I have a profound gratefulness to my yoga teacher, who made healthy light of the Covid-19 virus from the beginning. This set me on my way to freedom from anxiety, at least in the start of the race. His teachings in meditation with mantras helped tremendously with my lungs and inspired my heart to be in balance with a greater spirit than myself. In the darkest night, I knew who to call to come as the protector-destroyer. My yoga teacher had taught all his students this Hindu mantra and special prayer for Covid-19. We were doing it on a daily basis. As hard as it was for me to imagine doing a small ceremony daily, I managed to accomplish this powerful commitment. Thanks to his training and innovative methods, he eased my mind while building up my protective spiritual armour.

After every meditation, I was renewed. I have been alone, but never lonely. My solitude grew into solace. My heart has opened in a way I cannot describe with words. I had been grappling with this concept over the past two decades studying yoga seriously, but I suppose there is no better way to know thyself than to go to battle. During this Covid illness I literally had to fight my own mind and body and upgrade my Soul to meet the challenge.

I could say, although traumatic, it has been the best thing that ever happened to me. Thank GOD I passed the test. I am grateful to all who have been on the side lines waiting for me to pass the finish line of the marathon. One time someone told me the secret to finishing a marathon; "Make sure you have your boss at the last leg of the race, because he/she is the only one who can make you finish for sure!" My yoga teacher was there at the end telling me to do fast yoga and breathe loudly. I am positive it made a great difference in my full recovery to rid me of the last bits of virus between my lungs and my heart. That advice made me a sure winner! Thank goodness I listened!

Lastly, I would love to thank the birds and the stars that made every day so lovely! It was a small gesture from the Cosmos that had a great impact on the start of my day (early mornings). I am ever so grateful for my eyes and ears. Elephants have big ears, long memories and guard their strength only for essential battles. For we all could learn from these great beings. In the silence I grew stronger. The essence of flowers came alive. True BEAUTY revealed her enigma, it was there in the valley that always was...in my own Soul.

This virus attack taught me to be FEARLESS.
I will never be the same. I am STRONGER from this ordeal.
Truly, I learned my Mind, Body & Soul can carry me through LIFE.

OM Shanti Shanti Shanti OM

42

Introducción de autor (español)

Retrospectiva 2020. ¡Navegando aguas inexploradas!

A principios de la primavera de marzo, me encontré en medio de una pandemia y sin saberlo en un epicentro en Madrid, España. Ahora me doy cuenta de que muchos de los que no han estado en contacto con el Covid-19 personalmente parecen sentir que es un misterio que esté por ahí en alguna parte. Supongo que yo tendría la misma impresión si las circunstancias se hubieran desarrollado de forma diferente. De hecho, hasta el 8 de marzo, recuerdo haber pensado que Italia estaba exagerando al cancelar la marcha del Dia de la Mujer como me transmitió una amiga, residente cerca de Milán. Tres días después, el 11 de marzo, Madrid estaba iniciando su cierre. Recuerdo que iba en el tren de cercanías y todo el mundo estaba charlando sobre el repentino anuncio del Gobierno de cerrar las escuelas en 24h. Al bajar del tren y entrar en la estación, noté que la gente se movía con un propósito. Se me ocurrió que era pertinente llegar a casa y coger el carro de la compra y dirigirse a la tienda. Nos venció como una ola de calor en un pequeño pueblo polvoriento del sur de España, una pesada e insoportable presión que aumenta a cada hora que pasa. En este punto me sentía perfectamente bien. La tienda de comestibles estaba llena de gente con grandes cantidades de alimentos, provisiones y papel higiénico. Tenía mi pequeño carro y sólo podía llevar lo que entraba en él con una bolsa en mi hombro como reserva. Era una tarde soleada y agradable, así que aproveché el buen tiempo para ir a dar un paseo en bicicleta. Los días en primavera pueden ser muy cambiantes y estábamos saliendo de un período de frío, así que aproveché la brisa cálida para distraerme.

La auto cuarentena me golpeó como una bofetada en la cara.
¿Cómo pude pasar de pedalear en mi bicicleta a estar postrada en mi cama en 24horas?

Estoy muy agradecida por el contacto continuo con mi familia, amigos, y mis consejeros médicos (oeste y este) al haber sido capaces de ayudarme en una recuperación confinada en el hogar evitando la hospitalización. La auto-cuarentena significa aislamiento y cuidado completo por sí mismo. Tengo que admitir que los años de entrenamiento de yoga y disciplina dados a una edad temprana me ayudaron enormemente a mantener mi cerebro en blanco, incluso cuando no estaba respondiendo por falta de oxígeno o hinchazón. Las noticias de Wuhan también ayudaron a poner el virus en perspectiva, especialmente un informe de un residente británico en el extranjero que informó que había tenido un resfriado un día y de repente cayó enfermo con neumonía y fue llevado de urgencia al hospital con complicaciones respiratorias. Finalmente admití mi fiebre después de ese encantador paseo en bicicleta alrededor del río y el atracón de compras. Ahora pienso en lo afortunada que fui al preparar mi casa con suministros que tendrían que durarme tres semanas. En realidad, sólo había pensado en frutas y verduras frescas para 10 días para aguantar el encierro original programado por el gobierno. Sin embargo, me abastecí de frijoles, arroz y sardinas por si acaso duraba más días recordando otras emergencias. Tan pronto como me di cuenta de que tenía fiebre el viernes 13' estaba postrada en la cama con un dolor insoportable de riñones y piernas. Rápidamente me deshidraté y me debilité tanto que ni siquiera pude planear una comida, así que sólo me abstuve de realizar cualquier esfuerzo. Amigos míos me aconsejaron evitar la aspirina y tratar de luchar contra mi propio sistema inmunológico. Esto estaba en línea con mi propia filosofía sobre la enfermedad, así que le ayudé. Los informes eran dispares sobre el resultado de los medicamentos derivados de la aspirina, así que lo soporté s siguientes 5 días sola con el virus en mi apartamento. En este punto, era inevitable, tuve que imponerme una auto-cuarentena durante 14 días, incluso después de que la fiebre disminuyera. A su vez, comencé a racionar mi comida y papel higiénico.

De capullo a mariposa.
Te invito a mi viaje de metamorfosis.

Comencé este viaje en un tren que iba desde Madrid, una importante capital europea y epicentro de Covid-19 a un pueblo rural cercano. Después de vivir en varias capitales urbanas de todo el mundo, llenas de desafíos vibrantes y nuevas experiencias (Tokio, Bangkok, San Francisco, etc.), un pequeño virus me abrió los ojos de forma más clara y rápida que cualquier otra situación a la que me había enfrentado en mi vida. Era un nuevo tren bala con su propio transcurso del tiempo rápido hacia adelante, y me aferraba a la barandilla jadeando por aire a su paso por un túnel oscuro. Sentí como si me dirigiera hacia el abismo, como una historia interminable. Mi cuerpo era su patio de recreo y no tenía control sobre dónde atacaría. Sólo tuve que subirme a la ola, una ola de calor, seca y polvorienta. Empecé a escribir este libro de poesía por dos razones: 1) terapia de recuperación para plasmar mis pensamientos en papel para captar la experiencia y 2) para ofrecer aliento a otros para afrontar el virus en casa sin hospitalización.

El resultado de este viaje fue la transición de una urbanita a una agricultora orgánica a tiempo parcial. Literalmente no tengo ningún deseo de pisar un centro urbano y francamente me asusta, ya que asocio la vida de la ciudad con riesgos para la salud. Estoy segura de que esto es una reacción a una dura realidad y puede cambiar en el futuro. Sin embargo, me pareció que anhelaba sol y aire fresco después del calvario que duró aproximadamente 6 semanas. Mi masa muscular bajó tremendamente y perdí casi 9 kilos (20 libras) en 3 semanas. Tuve que volver a aprender a caminar y recuperar fuerzas en todos mis órganos. Luego tuve que volver a aprender a comer para mantenerme en mi peso "ideal". Fue uno de los efectos secundarios positivos. Alquilé una parcela de tierra para iniciar un jardín después de encontrar las plantas como fuente de consuelo en la soleada terraza trasera de mi apartamento durante la cuarentena. El silencio era la mejor manera de recuperarse y los niveles de ruido se redujeron mucho durante el confinamiento. Estoy segura de que con tés ayurvédicos durante el virus y yoga pranayama para la recuperación, combinado con estar en contacto con la naturaleza, puede influir claramente a cualquier persona que se enfrenta a este tipo de virus u otra amenaza de la vida.

Mis alas de mariposa han surgido de un estado de cristalización, estoy agradecida.

43

Mi aprendizaje (español)

Introducción

Este viaje a través del cuerpo, la mente y el alma fue una sorpresa para mí. Me gustaría transmitir algunos consejos útiles a la hora de lidiar con este virus de película y el impacto que tuvo personalmente en mí. En Madrid hubo diversas reacciones al virus, de leves a mortales. Yo estuve en la mitad de este rango. Algunos amigos tuvieron versiones leves con síntomas gripales que duraban una semana aproximadamente con pérdida de olor y sabor (indicador principal de Covid-19). Yo experimenté en mi cuerpo un recorrido completo de los síntomas del virus, con desafíos en cada paso del camino. He intentado recordar los aspectos más destacados que podrían ser útiles, ampliados con mis notas junto a la cama durante las 5 semanas. Mi práctica espiritual ha evolucionado del Oeste al Este con un toque de Nativa Americana expresada en el respeto por la Tierra, la práctica de yoga y el amor en acción. Este virus fue sin duda el "embaucador" Coyote empujándome a cavar profundamente para enfrentarme al Gran Espíritu; física, emocional y espiritualmente. Listo o no, venía, y no se escondía. Era como una búsqueda de visión interior, vagando a través de mi propio organismo hasta el nivel celular. Jugaba con mi cerebro a través de la deshidratación y me obligó a bajar la velocidad como una serpiente en el calor del desierto. En el peor de los casos, no tuve otra opción que renunciar a la vida como ser humano independiente bajo control. Finalmente me fusioné con la Naturaleza, y abrí mi corazón a un nuevo capítulo en la vida.

Entiendo que usted puede que nunca caiga enfermo con este virus, pero tal vez un ser querido lo padezca. Con suerte, con mi relato usted puede que sea capaz de entender sus síntomas y ayudarle. Mi intención es alertar al público de la velocidad de este virus, ya que ataca el sistema humano, lo que deja muy poco tiempo para reaccionar. Por lo tanto, este libro ha sido creado para la prevención, la advertencia sincera, y retrospectiva 2020. Estoy agradecida por la información de las redes sociales que me dieron una idea de la voracidad del virus, que a su vez me puso en alerta desde el principio explicado por un hombre británico en Wuhan que se estaba recuperando del virus. Tuvo un resfriado, luego pasó rápidamente a neumonía y poco después fue hospitalizado. Teniendo en cuenta el impacto de su relato del virus, tomé todos los síntomas como serios y cualquier cambio como peligrosamente cerca de la línea de hospitalización.

Al principio, pude mantenerme al día con mis meditaciones y yoga. El yoga físico se dejó una vez que era obvio que mis pulmones estaban debilitados y necesitaba permanecer menos activa en la cama. Sin embargo, continué sesiones de meditación de 30 minutos con mantras (cantando) y pranayama (respirando) todos los días para ayudar a mantener los pulmones en una mínima forma. Muchos días me estremecí ya que apenas podía hacerlos, pero continué la práctica. Me sorprende que pudiera reunir la energía para hacer esas sesiones, cuando todo parecía "misión imposible". Parecía comida para el alma y esencial para mi bienestar general. Tuve que tener cuidado con la duración por razones de energía y calculé mi relación de ingesta de alimentos con respecto a la digestión para obtener resultados óptimos. (Por ejemplo, tenía cuatro horas de liberación lenta de energía después de comer avena para el desayuno).

Mi actitud mental fue vital para mantener todo equilibrado y me fue de utilidad el conocimiento general de mi cuerpo a raíz de enfermedades anteriores. Creo que mi actitud marcó la fina línea que me separaba de la línea de meta en casa o en un hospital. Uno fácilmente puede introducirse en una espiral negativa hundiendo el sistema inmunológico con estrés emocional si uno deja la mente sin control. Tuve suerte de haber recibido una alerta temprana de mi profesor de yoga, que me mantuvo riendo durante la primera etapa. Mantuve esta actitud solicitando chistes para impulsar mi sistema inmunológico. España fue un flujo constante de chistes que venían de todas partes con vídeos caseros e imágenes que parecían interminables junto con otros mensajes. Me concentré en la ligereza de la risa, solo, pero eficaz.

La disciplina fue otra cualidad que resultó vital. Necesité mucha atención para mantener una rutina (diseñada para cumplir con cada fase). Significó atención plena para moverse lentamente y mantenerse enfocada en las tareas a través de cada proceso y adaptarse a todos los cambios en mi reacción corporal al virus. Me alegro de haber sido entrenada primero por mis estrictos padres de la juventud. Durante los últimos 25 años ese entrenamiento fue seguido por un maestro de yoga con un carácter estricto. La singularidad de mi profesor de yoga es su profundo don para bromear cuando los tiempos son difíciles, como Covid-19, y su actitud positiva para enfrentar los desafíos de salud. También utiliza Ayurveda (antigua filosofía medicinal india) para hacer frente al bienestar general del cuerpo directamente a través de alimentos, hierbas y meditación. Me dieron recetas para combinar en mi dieta para impulsar el sistema inmunológico y mantener mi cuerpo a salvo de los ataques del virus a los órganos y al sistema respiratorio. Meditación que había aprendido a lo largo de los años y practicaba a diario.

Mi sorpresa fue el viaje espiritual, que fue más allá de mis expectativas, y que no tiene precio. Ha tenido un efecto duradero. Tendría que admitir que los avances del viaje de mi alma fueron una bendición como resultado de esta experiencia. Fue la tranquilidad de la enfermedad (por el aislamiento y el bajo oxígeno) lo que me permitió profundamente eliminar la cubierta de ilusión de este escenario tangible del mundo "real" y enfrentar lo intangible, mi Creador. Llegó de la manera más creativa con amor, risas y belleza. Me fusioné con la lluvia y floté en las plumas de los cantos de los pájaros, mientras caía en un sueño profundo. Encontré el camino donde la belleza habita en el Alma.

La recuperación es más difícil de lo que uno puede imaginar y uno debe ser consciente de que este virus permanece si no se trata correctamente. Tan pronto como estuve lista para el ejercicio y la actividad física, comencé la rutina sugerida por el médico. Fue lento, pero constante. Entonces mi corazón empezó a molestarme, así pensé. Le pregunté al doctor, un cirujano del corazón. Indicó que era normal sentir presión en el corazón con la menor capacidad de los pulmones. Luego le pedí una rutina específica a mi profesor de yoga para el corazón y los pulmones. Me alertó para expulsar el virus de los pulmones con una técnica especial de yoga aeróbico. Creo que es esencial tratar el período de recuperación seriamente, a fin de superar el virus completamente sin efectos duraderos o recaídas. La siguiente es una síntesis de las lecciones aprendidas. Este virus comenzó a mostrar síntomas el viernes, 13 de marzo.

Cuerpo:

Durante el virus y la recuperación. Los estudios mencionados en esta sección fueron investigados después de la recuperación y se citan en la sección de referencia.

Fiebre: La fiebre era una fiebre baja que nunca alcanzaba altas temperaturas, ni experimenté escalofríos. Fue molesto porque duró más de lo que suelen durar mis fiebres habituales ya que estuvo conmigo durante una semana. Además, al principio pasó casi desapercibida. Por lo tanto, hacía mi vida sin prestar atención a su inicio. Después del primer día decidí no tomar aspirinas ni antinflamatorios. Me advirtieron de que podían empeorar mi condición, así que apliqué remedios tradicionales, principalmente dormir, descansar, sonreír y soportarlo. Controlé mi temperatura de forma regular para informar a mi médico más tarde. Era molesto, ya que perduró. La paciencia es una virtud perfeccionada por la experiencia. Nunca había tenido ese tipo de fiebre. En el pasado, por lo general podía sobrellevarla con un par de aspirinas e ir a trabajar.

Recuperación: Tengo cuidado de no sobrecalentarme o coger frío que pueda desencadenar una fiebre. Me mantengo alejada del sol al mediodía y me aseguro de llevar una bufanda para las brisas de la mañana temprano. Soy más cautelosa con los cambios extremos de temperatura que pueden afectar a mi cuerpo.

Riñón: Después de la aparición de la fiebre, me empezaron a doler los riñones y el dolor evolucionó hacia un sufrimiento insoportable después del tercer día. Estaba contraída como una pelota en la cama con sensaciones insoportables como de un cuchillo apuñalando la parte baja de mi espalda y mis piernas. Duró 5 días junto con la baja fiebre. ¡Mi nivel de deshidratación fue increíble! Mantenía dos termos grandes junto a mi cama con agua tibia (no se recomienda agua fría) y los rellenaba constantemente. ¡Nunca parecía suficiente agua, y sin embargo sorprendentemente no estaba eliminando los líquidos! No tenía escalofríos y no sudaba. Me quedé sorprendida por esta reacción. La proporción de agua ingerida con respecto a las visitas al baño era completamente "novedosa" y no encajaba en mi esquema de normalidad. Normalmente al cabo de una hora, después de beber líquidos estaría visitando el baño. En esta situación no necesitaba ir al baño. Perdí la cuenta de mi proceso de eliminación, pero noté que era muy bajo. Adonde iba el agua, no tengo ni idea.

Mi profesor de yoga me sugirió cúrcuma, pimienta negra y bebida caliente de jengibre, y los tomé en polvo (bio) disueltos en agua caliente a lo largo de todo el virus para el riñón y el hígado. Probé a tomar esta mezcla temprano en la mañana, pero era demasiado fuerte para mi estómago. Cambié a la opción de mediodía, ya que utilicé la mezcla como base para sopas para ahorrar tiempo y acabar tareas. Acabo de beber la mezcla (cúrcuma, pimienta negra y jengibre) primero y luego añadí agua con ajo y otras hierbas como tomillo o comino. Finalmente, las verduras para la sopa. El ajo picado y hervido liberó a sus agentes antibacterianos y funcionó bien de acuerdo a Ayurveda. La cúrcuma y el jengibre ayudaron a las células del hígado y riñones para que se enfrenten al desafío del virus. Esta combinación también fue buena para los pulmones (agentes antiinflamatorios).

Encontré estudios que apoyaron este remedio Ayurveda en las siguientes declaraciones:

- “La cúrcuma, una especia que ha sido reconocida durante mucho tiempo por sus propiedades medicinales, ha llamado el interés tanto del mundo médico / científico como de los entusiastas culinarios, ya que es la principal fuente de la curcumina polifenol. Ayuda en el manejo de condiciones oxidativas e inflamatorias, síndrome metabólico, artritis, ansiedad, e hiperlipidemia.”
- “También puede ayudar en el manejo de la inflamación in-

ducida por el ejercicio y dolor muscular, mejorando así la recuperación y el rendimiento en personas activas. Además, una dosis relativamente baja de la mezcla puede proporcionar beneficios para la salud de las personas que no tienen problemas de salud diagnosticados. La mayoría de estos beneficios se pueden atribuir a sus efectos antioxidantes y antiinflamatorios."

- "Ingerir la curcumina por sí mismo no conduce a los beneficios asociados para la salud debido a su mala biodisponibilidad, que parece ser principalmente debido a la mala absorción, rápido metabolismo y rápida eliminación. Hay varios componentes que pueden aumentar la biodisponibilidad. Por ejemplo, piperina es el principal componente activo de la pimienta negra y, cuando se combina en un complejo con curcumina, se ha demostrado que puede aumentar la biodisponibilidad un 2000%."

Recuperación: Todavía me voy a la cama con 2 botellas grandes de agua tibia junto a mi cama. Una la lleno con agua tibia de limón para beber al despertarme, y la otra la lleno con agua normal o té de hierbas. Bebo zumo de limón caliente (hecho la noche anterior y puesto junto a mi cama en un termo) para beber al comienzo del día con el fin de activar la bilis del hígado. Lleva tiempo cambiar a alcalino, por eso lo bebo de inmediato en la cama. Comencé con algunos tés de hierbas locales como diente de León y cola de caballo (bio) para rejuvenecer el hígado y los riñones respectivamente. Sigo con cúrcuma, jengibre y pimienta negra para fortalecer mi hígado y riñones. Presto mucha atención a mi ingesta de líquidos, mínimo 8 vasos al día con el estómago vacío, entre comidas alternadas con infusiones.

Nódulos linfáticos: La sobrecarga de células muertas en los ganglios linfáticos hizo que se obstruyeran. Esto dio lugar a que mis piernas entrasen en una inquietante agonía de pinchazos Me despertaba por la noche debido al dolor a lo largo de mis piernas desde todos los ángulos. Me levantaba y bailaba, las ponía en algo, pero era en vano. Finalmente, recordé a mi profesor de yoga explicando una limpieza linfática para aplicar en la piel. Hice un exfoliante linfático casero para mi piel elaborado a partir de especias disponibles en la cocina como semillas de mostaza, arroz rojo, canela, jengibre, comino. Lo froté por todo mi cuerpo y lo desempolvé en el baño (desastre). Luego apliqué yogur calmante en mi piel seguido de una ducha caliente. ¡Me aliviaba!

Empecé a prestar atención a la limpieza más a fondo de mi piel de forma rutinaria (como un exfoliante japonés antes del baño) para eliminar las toxinas. Hacía un lavado extra en la ducha como rutina diaria, no importa lo sucio que me sintiera. Era vital mantener esta rutina en la mañana después del desayuno para que mi cuerpo se liberara de las toxinas acumuladas en la piel. Los exfoliantes linfáticos se convirtieron en un ritual semanal añadido al desafío del virus.

Recuperación: Continúo frotando bien mi piel en cada ducha. Me doy más duchas para eliminar las toxinas en la piel, especialmente después de despertarme, de realizar actividad física y antes de acostarme. Mantengo mis especias abastecidas para exfoliantes linfáticos y yogur como toque final para calmar la piel.

Hígado: Irónicamente, he sido consciente de mi hígado cuando tomaba píldoras contra la malaria mientras trabajé en un campo de refugiados en Tailandia (a veces citado como un remedio Covid-19). Desconocedora de su principal ingrediente y de su efecto a largo plazo, debilitó mi hígado hasta el punto del agotamiento y mareos. Me llevó 14 años recuperarme. Por suerte, el hígado es un órgano que rejuvenece. Me di cuenta cuando mi hígado fue atacado por este virus principalmente debido a la repentina y extrema falta de energía. Me sentí como si me hubieran atropellado 10 camiones. Agregué una dosis de cúrcuma (soluble en grasa) a mi yogur sabiendo que el potente remedio Ayurveda aumentaría la vitalidad hepática como un contraataque al virus.

Encontré estudios que explicaban los efectos positivos de la cúrcuma en el hígado en las siguientes declaraciones:

- "Hay varios mecanismos plausibles que sugieren un efecto favorable de la curcumina en la función hepática. Estudios han indicado que el estrés oxidativo y el trastorno del sistema inmunitario desempeñan un papel importante en contribuir a la disfunción hepática como NAFLD.35 En este caso, la curcumina puede mejorar el estrés oxidativo y prevenir el NAFLD mediante la disminución de la producción de especies reactivas de oxígeno, la expresión de proteína hepática del estrés oxidativo, citoquinas proinflamatorias y quimio quinas tales como interferón (IFN), interleucina-1 y proteína inducible IFN 10.36, 37."
- "Estudios basados en células han demostrado el potencial de la cúrcuma como un antimicrobiano, insecticida, larvicida, anti mutagénico, radio protector, y agente anticancerígeno. La cúrcuma también se ha utilizado para apoyar la función hepática y para tratar la ictericia en la medicina herbaria ayurvédica y china."
- "La investigación durante la última década ha identificado numerosas entidades químicas de la cúrcuma, y la ciencia moderna ha proporcionado una base lógica en la seguridad y eficacia de la cúrcuma contra las enfermedades humanas. Los datos epidemiológicos indican que algunos cánceres extremadamente comunes en el mundo occidental son mucho menos frecuentes en las regiones (Sudeste Asiático, por ejemplo) donde la cúrcuma se consume de forma generalizada en la dieta. Esta especia se ha encontrado que es bien tolerada en dosis de gramo en seres humanos. La cúrcuma dietética contiene más de 300 componentes diferentes. "

Además, comí tantos alimentos amargos como me fue posible durante el proceso, como alcachofas cultivadas localmente y espárragos. Los alimentos amargos también son útiles para el hígado.

Recuperación: Mi experiencia previa para rejuvenecer mi hígado fue beber 1 litro de té de hierbas de diente de León a lo largo del día, extendiéndolo desde la mañana hasta la tarde. En el caso del virus, ha sido bastante útil aplicar el mismo remedio. Alterné dos infusiones para la recuperación de hígado y riñón (diente de león y cola de caballo) en semanas alternas. Me imagino que las tomaré durante 3 meses para recuperar completamente el hígado y el riñón. Por lo tanto, he evitado el café durante el virus y durante este período de recuperación. Ejerce demasiada presión sobre estos órganos debilitados.

Digestión: Viajar por Asia ha sido una hoja de doble filo con destacadas lecciones de desafíos gastrointestinales y sabiduría ancestral para el tracto digestivo. Por un lado, aprendí a aniquilar al virus o bacterias, inducidos problemas digestivos, a base de arroz blanco. Curiosamente, acababa de comprar un poco de arroz blanco orgánico (debido a la falta de arroz integral) y lo tuve disponible de forma fácil durante las primeras semanas del virus. Observé el extraño hedor y la coloración de mis deposiciones, sin comparación con otras enfermedades.

En cualquier caso, estaba demasiado enferma para realmente preocuparme. Había perdido la mayor parte de mi olfato y sabor, pero curiosamente esto era notablemente potente. En realidad, no tenía diarrea, pero estaba lo suficientemente suelta como para no ser normal. Observé los cambios y tomé notas sobre las complicaciones dietéticas. Empecé a notar que el aceite y las verduras crudas eran problemáticos, así que los eliminé, incluso el aceite de oliva de alta calidad. Cocí o hice al vapor mi comida. Para los aceites, sólo utilicé mantequilla bio en las tostadas y añadí un surtido rico en nueces a mis desayunos de avena y tentempiés de mediodía durante las actividades (trabajo físico o mental). Evité ensaladas o verduras crudas, y cociné todo. Esto mantuvo mi bazo saludable al reducir los alimentos acuosos al mínimo y resultó evitar su inflamación. Frutas crudas en el desayuno, media mañana antes del yoga y a la hora de acostarse (bananas). Era vital mantener mi cuerpo en el lado seco, por lo que estas tres raciones de fruta durante todo el día fueron suficientes para equilibrar mi dieta en cuanto a la fibra y los minerales.

Recordé que la avena era buena para la desintoxicación en las dietas de recuperación de la quimio contra el cáncer que utilizaron amigos. Cambié mis porciones de comida para no sobrecargar el sistema digestivo y las extendí un poco para dar tiempo a la digestión. A los cítricos (limón, naranja, kiwi) les di 20 minutos de digestión con el fin de hacer la transición de ácido a alcalino y así producir un sistema inmunológico fuerte. (Nunca se toman con productos lácteos, incluida la vitamina C). Eliminé todos los lácteos para no obstruir el sistema linfático, excepto un yogur al día. Necesitaba los probióticos para reconstruir el proceso digestivo.

Recuperación: Continué con poco o ningún lácteo (un poco de leche con té de jengibre y un yogur). Esperé 3 meses para reintroducir la ensalada en mi dieta. Empecé con un poco de lechuga y pepino (bueno para contrarrestar los alimentos ácidos). Continúe con porciones pequeñas. Continué espaciando proteínas y verduras para dar tiempo a la digestión de cada grupo de alimentos. Por ejemplo, después del yoga tomo proteína y luego me ducho. Es el tiempo suficiente para permitir que el estómago se concentre sólo en la digestión de la proteína antes de sobrecargarlo con el siguiente grupo de verduras. Trato de masticar a fondo cada alimento para dar al estómago la señal de las glándulas salivales de liberar la enzima apropiada para ayudar a la digestión adecuada. Comencé antes del almuerzo con un aperitivo de yogur lassi (sin azúcar o miel) que es simplemente una mezcla de cuatro de agua por una de yogur para crear el original "buttermilk". La cúrcuma y la bebida de pimienta negra se añadió a este aperitivo para preparar el estómago para mi comida principal.

Pulmones: En un punto (2 semanas) empecé a darme cuenta de que mis pulmones tenían una sensación extraña. Clínicamente, se llamaría "falta de aliento". Poéticamente, sólo puedo describirlo como una ventana abierta en la mitad inferior de mis pulmones. Tal vez esta forma de nombrarlo desde el punto de vista poético le restaba gravedad. Sin embargo, para mí eso fue un punto de inflexión para modificar drásticamente mi actividad porque no mejoró después de unos días. De hecho, empeoró. Creo que fue una combinación de negación del síntoma y la gestión de la crisis lo que hizo darle menos atención a este síntoma. Como parte del plan nacional de salud Covid-19, se nos había dado la posibilidad de llamar a un número de teléfono especial disponible 24/7 para solicitar atención médica en casa o una ambulancia para ir al hospital. Mi dificultad para respirar fue la razón principal para hacer esa llamada. Supongo que no estaba lista para rendirme, así que intenté usar como remedio el descanso en cama. Me retrotrajo al cine en blanco y negro de niña cuando los personajes se quedaban en la cama durmiendo para luchar contra la enfermedad.

Detuve toda actividad no esencial y sólo hice uso de la mañana para el desayuno, la ducha, la meditación y cocinar el almuerzo. Cada actividad la hacía de forma lenta y calculada. Día a día me di cuenta de mi incapacidad para contener la respiración en mis ejercicios diarios de respiración de yoga (pranayama). Me reía de mi forma de hacer los ejercicios y me di cuenta de que el virus había afectado a mis pulmones. Dejé de realizar todo el yoga físico. A las 2-3pm estaba en la cama. Me sentaba en la cama con almohadas para mantenerme erguida con el fin de mantener las vías respiratorias abiertas. Empecé a leer en línea revistas literarias con poesía o cortometrajes que nunca tuve tiempo de disfrutar. Encontré en una estantería un viejo libro que me regaló mi mejor amigo que nunca tuve tiempo de leer. Escondida dentro había una dulce nota. Fue casi el primer libro que encontré y fue perfecto. Un estilo poético de cuentos escritos el siglo pasado por Kahlil Gibran, autor del *Profeta*, con un ritmo lento.

Empecé a preocuparme a medida que pasaban los días. Mi médico estaba preocupado y me contactaba más a menudo. Mentalmente, estaba llegando al límite. Analicé mi vida preguntándome si realmente la había completado lo suficiente. ¿Había contribuido lo suficiente a la sociedad? Además, me preguntaba si para aliviar mis pulmones, vapor de agua con una toalla sobre la estufa era un buen método o no. Resultó no ser un buen remedio. Sin alivio. De hecho, no tenía ni congestión ni agua. Un amigo me sugirió un remedio simple, que era hacer gárgaras con vinagre de sidra de manzana y, también, tragar un poco. Hice eso y me pareció que ayudaba junto con el resto. Tuve suerte de encontrar vinagre de sidra de manzana bio en el supermercado del barrio. ¡Había muchos artículos agotados, pero estaba el vinagre que necesitaba! Había cogido una botella pensando que sería bueno tener a mano para el encierro. (También encontré cúrcuma fresca en el antiguo mercado, un artículo raro. Nunca lo volví a ver después de abril). Una suerte increíble.

Esta fase duró fácilmente 2 semanas. Controlé mi capacidad de respiración intentándome arrodillar por la mañana al aire fresco de mi balcón. En mi práctica de pranayama tomé nota de cuánto podía hacer antes de necesitar tomar aire. Parecía una eternidad antes de que pudiera arrodillarme o hacer al menos el 50% de mi pranayama. Sólo tenía que ser paciente. Estaba tan cansada de estar cansada. Familiares, amigos y compañeros de yoga estaban constantemente ahí en las redes sociales para alentar mi actitud positiva y se conectaban varias veces al día, especialmente mi amiga de Italia. Parecía saber exactamente lo que estaba experimentando, ya que la pandemia estaba asolando el norte de Italia al mismo tiempo. No podía hablar, demasiada energía. Nunca tuve tos en sí misma. Sólo tuve un montón de carraspeo seco. ¡Me alegré el día que pude arrodillarme en mi balcón al amanecer! ¡Empecé a saludar al sol todos los días con mis nuevos pulmones! ¡Recordé el día que pude bailar! 21 de abril.

La fase que permanecí semi-encamada para combatir el virus en mis pulmones fue devastadora para los músculos de mis piernas. Tuve que volver a aprender a caminar. Mi cerebro también se vio afectado con inflamación y, sin embargo, tuve un hermoso efecto secundario de tipo espiritual en esos momentos de semi consciencia.

Recuperación: Después de 5 semanas estaba tan agotada del virus dado su curso alrededor de mi cuerpo, especialmente el último ataque a mis pulmones. Cuando remitió, fue como bajar de una nave espacial de vuelta a la Tierra. Empecé a sentir el deseo de hacer ejercicio. Surgieron preguntas sobre cuánto. Mi doctor me envió un plan de recuperación. Dado el susto con los pulmones, tuve mucho cuidado con el ejercicio. Empecé con rutinas lentas de brazo y pierna sugeridas por el volante del fisioterapeuta. Parecía patético para una persona atlética como yo. Sin embargo, yo era consciente de mis límites y, en realidad, estaba en modo de cuidado personal para tratarme de forma delicada. En ese momento tuve una presión cardíaca que fue preocupante. Otro síntoma de Covid-19 que envía a las personas al hospital. Consulté a un amigo médico, un cirujano del corazón que se encargaba del seguimiento de pacientes de Covid-19, para preguntarle sobre mi situación. Me aseguró que era normal dada la menor capacidad del pulmón. Así que estaba más tranquila.

Luego consulté a mi profesor de yoga. Estaba en este modo de recuperación súper lento y cuidadoso. Quería un poco del dulce yoga Hatha (posiciones relajantes) para el corazón. Su sugerencia me dejó de una pieza. Dijo: "Haz yoga rápido y respira fuerte por la boca". Tuve que confirmar su mensaje de texto. Nos había estado enseñando la técnica de "respirar fuego" durante los últimos dos años, llamada Bhastika. Su Kundalini Tantra Yoga es una combinación de momento (principalmente regiones pélvicas y de hombros) con liberación de aliento para bloqueos emocionales en el cuerpo. Apenas podía caminar, así que ahora "yoga rápido". Me explicó que el virus podría estar bloqueado entre el corazón y el pulmón y era vital expulsarlo para evitar efectos persistentes. Nunca se ha equivocado en 25 años, así que lo hice.

Hice mi propia rutina de 12 minutos de yoga aeróbico basado en sus técnicas de movimientos de cadera y hombro con respiración exagerada para expulsar el virus. Usé mi bicicleta como calentamiento o compras de comestibles con los 3 tramos de escaleras para trabajar el sudor antes de hacer este yoga. Comí fruta (kiwi) justo antes para darme un empuje de energía y esperé 15 minutos para su digestión. Entonces, puse mi cronómetro y comencé este "novedoso" enfoque. ¡Funcionó! Me hice más fuerte día tras día.

Cerebro: Los niveles de oxígeno se agotaron significativamente debido a la menor capacidad pulmonar y mi cerebro era menos funcional. Me dormía más fácilmente en esas tardes y no podía concentrarme. De hecho, comencé a entrar en un extraño modo de consciencia. El mundo material comenzó a importarme cada vez menos. Los días de estar en la cama por las tardes se fusionaron en un solo momento.

Antes de contraer el virus, trabajaba sin parar, viajando a Madrid la mayoría de los días por la mañana temprano y regresando tarde por la noche. Los fines de semana, solía mirar mi habitación con la hermosa luz brillando a través de las cortinas de encaje en la ventana sur con el deseo de hacer una siesta. En ese momento no tenía tiempo extra para tanta frivolidad. Tenía que ponerme al día con las tareas domésticas, ir de compras y prepararme para la semana con el lavado. Parecía una broma que me hacía Dios. El Covid-19 había convertido mi dormitorio en un cuarto de bebé para largas siestas de tarde. (*Tenga cuidado con lo que desea*).

La inflamación del cerebro, hasta donde confirmar, es normal en algunos pacientes. Tenía que acostarme con la cabeza sobre el costado de la cama para dejar que la sangre fluyera hacia mi cerebro como método de alivio. No podía hablar más de 30 minutos. Al comienzo del ataque del virus, tuve un fuerte dolor de cabeza con un episodio de fiebre. Más tarde se convirtió en un estado mental de languidez general con la fase pulmonar. No podía trabajar en línea más de una hora seguida o hacer tareas en mi ordenador. Limité toda actividad mental a un mínimo.

Consulté a mi médico, quien me aseguró que era normal dados los niveles de oxígeno y el estado emocional del confinamiento en mi cuerpo. Ella me insistió en que me asegurase de que la casa se mantenía bien ventilada y en que saliese a tomar aire fresco. Ella estaba segura de que mejoraría con la actividad al aire libre.

Recuperación: ¡El 2 de mayo pudimos hacer ejercicio al aire libre! ¡Qué día para regocijarse! Monté en bicicleta a lo largo de los caminos rurales arbolados con los pájaros en los campos disfrutando de la primavera tardía. (Gracias a Dios que había comprado una bicicleta justo antes del confinamiento). Fue muy difícil caminar debido al agotamiento de la masa muscular de las piernas. Mientras que montar en bicicleta era más fácil. ¡Montar en bicicleta por la mañana temprano fue tan maravilloso para mi cerebro y pulmones! Continué teniendo mucho cuidado de no sobrecargar mi cerebro. Seguí haciendo los ejercicios de yoga aeróbico y la respiración de fuego para aumentar la capacidad pulmonar. Ponía mi cabeza sobre el lado de la cama todas las noches durante unos minutos hasta que mi cerebro se sentía normal.

Además, para limpiar mis fosas nasales comencé a practicar la técnica de Ayurveda llamada "neti pot" (jala neti). Consiste en un lavado de las fosas nasales con agua tibia y sal. Mi profesor de yoga recomienda esta técnica una vez a la semana para eliminar las toxinas en forma de cristales que se acumulan en las fosas nasales y que es una de las causas del dolor de cabeza (cerebro). La práctica diaria de pranayama despeja las vías respiratorias y facilita este tipo de enjuague de las fosas nasales.

Alquilé una parcela de tierra física y mentalmente agradable con un montón de aire fresco y sol para trabajarla. ¡La naturaleza fue silenciosamente calmando mi estado mental y la agricultura me mantuvo centrada en una tarea con alegría! Era una extensión del minijardín de mi casa que había comenzado durante el encierro. Mi profesor de yoga también es agricultor en su tiempo libre y dice que la naturaleza siempre te da "amor". Era perfecto para sanar mi cerebro en una transición del estado de ensueño intangible al reino tangible.

Comencé este libro como una forma de volver a activar mi cerebro, pero de forma lenta. La poesía ha sido fácil para mí desde que era una niña, así que era una manera maravillosa de recuperarme. No me preocupé por demasiados detalles. Acabo de establecer un plan simple de 3 poemas para cada capítulo. Traté de hacerlo al mismo tiempo placentero y útil para las personas. Ha sido una experiencia mágica escribir este libro de un virus que me arrojó a un torbellino y mi cerebro al vacío.

Curiosamente, fue esta misma desconexión del cerebro la que ha provocado un nuevo camino en mi viaje espiritual (*Ver* sección Soul).

Médula ósea: Después de consultar varios estudios de Covid-19, encontré información útil sobre cómo el virus podría haber afectado mi médula ósea. Los glóbulos rojos y blancos se producen en la médula ósea junto con las plaquetas (células de coagulación de la sangre). Cuando este sistema es atacado o sobrecargado de trabajo, es ineficiente o no funciona. Por ejemplo, en algunos casos, aparecen coágulos sanguíneos en todos los órganos del cuerpo. Las células muertas o una proporción anormal de células inmaduras se acumulan en las glándulas linfáticas y en el bazo. No estoy segura exactamente de qué porcentaje de estas complicaciones experimenté, pero la baja energía (falta de glóbulos rojos) y los ganglios linfáticos sobrecargados (células muertas) fue evidente. Yo era consciente de estar alerta de cambios en el corazón, ya que eran signos mortales de alerta de complicaciones del virus (coágulos de sangre). Me di cuenta de que necesitaba ir a la cama temprano para evitar el agotamiento y, por lo general, mi energía no duraba más allá de las 19:00 pm. Me acostumbré a acostarme muy temprano. Ello implicaba que me levantaba antes, y con los pájaros cantando en mi ventana, era un placer. Parecía ser una parte natural de la vida.

Las siguientes declaraciones son de los estudios que encontré, y que me proporcionaron como resultado un conocimiento de la médula ósea:

- "Los coronavirus son capaces de infectar las células de la médula ósea, lo que resulta en hematopoyesis anormal. Hematopoyesis: La producción de todo tipo de células sanguíneas incluyendo su formación, desarrollo, y diferenciación de las células sanguíneas. La hematopoyesis es la producción de todos los componentes celulares de la sangre y el plasma sanguíneo. Se produce dentro del sistema hematopoyético, que incluye órganos y tejidos como la médula ósea, el hígado y el bazo. Simplemente, la hematopoyesis es el proceso a través del cual el cuerpo fabrica células sanguíneas. En los adultos, la hematopoyesis de glóbulos rojos y plaquetas ocurre principalmente en la médula ósea. En bebés y niños, también puede continuar en el bazo y el hígado."
- "Una baja suma de glóbulos blancos generalmente es causada por: Infecciones virales que interrumpen temporalmente el trabajo de la médula ósea."
- "Por lo general, una baja suma de glóbulos blancos significa que el cuerpo no está produciendo suficientes glóbulos blancos. Puede aumentar el riesgo de todo tipo de infecciones."
- "Algunos grupos, como las personas de ascendencia afrocaribeña y de Oriente Medio, a menudo tienen una baja suma de glóbulos blancos, pero esto es normal y no aumenta el riesgo de infecciones."
- "La médula ósea es el tejido que comprende la parte central de los huesos grandes. Los lechos capilares pulmonares dañados hacen que el proceso de ruptura de megacariocitos y liberación

plaquetaria se bloquee, lo que afecta a la liberación de las plaquetas en la circulación pulmonar e indirectamente conduce a una reducción de la síntesis plaquetaria en la circulación sistémica."

- "Los neutrófilos son la primera defensa contra los microorganismos invasores. El aumento de la susceptibilidad a patógenos comunes se ha atribuido generalmente a sumas extremadamente bajas (por debajo de 0,5 x 109/l) (13) y no se ha notificado que los individuos con sumas "bajas normales" o neutropenia étnica tengan un mayor riesgo, siempre y cuando los recuentos no disminuyan aún más. Sin embargo, en un estudio reciente se correlacionó de forma inversa la probabilidad de contraer tuberculosis de pacientes con enfermedades pulmonares abiertas con el recuento basal de neutrófilos en un estudio reciente."
- "La suma de neutrófilos en la sangre está determinada por la diferenciación y proliferación de células precursoras en la médula ósea, la liberación de neutrófilos maduros en la sangre, la marginación en órganos como el pulmón y el bazo, y la transmigración a través del revestimiento endotelial seguido de apoptosis de neutrófilos y la absorción por fagocitos. Un ejemplo es la neutropenia étnica benigna, que se encuentra en aproximadamente el 5% de los afroamericanos. Las reducidas y elevadas sumas de neutrófilos, incluso dentro del rango normal, se asocian con una mortalidad excesiva por todas las causas."
- "La médula ósea es donde se producen nuevas células sanguíneas. La médula ósea contiene dos tipos de células madre: hemopoyéticas (que pueden producir células sanguíneas) y estromales (que pueden producir grasa, cartílago y hueso). Existen dos tipos de médula ósea: la médula roja (también conocida como tejido mieloide) y la médula amarilla. Los glóbulos rojos, las plaquetas y la mayoría de los glóbulos blancos surgen en la médula roja; algunos glóbulos blancos se desarrollan en la mé-

dula amarilla. El color de la médula amarilla se debe al número mucho mayor de células grasas."

- "En los casos de pérdida grave de sangre, el cuerpo puede convertir la médula amarilla de nuevo en médula roja con el fin de aumentar la producción de células sanguíneas. La falta de glóbulos rojos hace que el cuerpo extraiga de la médula amarilla para convertirla de nuevo en médula roja para producir glóbulos rojos (portadores de oxígeno). La médula amarilla está diseñada para producir grasa y tejido a partir de los cinco años. La reducción de grasa y masa muscular resultante de inactividad (pérdida de masa muscular tras periodos encamado) y la falta de producción de la médula amarilla (células grasas) con el fin de ayudar a la médula roja arterial, produce glóbulos rojos sanos."
- "Los glóbulos rojos, los glóbulos blancos y las plaquetas se producen en la médula ósea roja. A medida que envejecemos, la distribución de la médula ósea roja y amarilla cambia. La mayor producción de la médula ósea en adultos se encuentra en las áreas del hombro, la pelvis y la columna vertebral de la estructura ósea del cuerpo humano."
- "Después de la producción de glóbulos blancos en la médula ósea, estas células necesitan moverse libremente para combatir la infección. Estas células circulan mejor por todo el cuerpo con la cabeza hacia abajo, y el tronco invertido en posiciones específicas de yoga. Los expertos en yoga recomiendan una postura de 'perro boca abajo'."
- "Nuestros cuerpos no producen vitamina C, pero la necesitamos para la función inmune, la estructura ósea, la absorción de hierro y la piel sana. Obtenemos vitamina C de nuestra dieta, generalmente en cítricos, fresas, verduras verdes y tomates."
- "El sueño juega un papel importante en el trabajo de reparación en el cuerpo humano. Hay evidencia sustancial de que el estrés debilita el sistema inmunológico y nos hace vulnerables a infecciones y enfermedades. la relación entre el

sueño y un sistema inmunitario saludable, y el daño que puede tener la falta de sueño. Mientras que más sueño no necesariamente evitará que te enfermes, escatimar en él podría afectar negativamente a tu sistema inmunológico. El sistema inmunitario entra en acción durante ese tiempo. El ritmo natural para la reparación es de 22:00 - 23:00."

Recuperación: La cúrcuma y el jengibre están llenos de hierro, que es necesario para producir glóbulos rojos y blancos. A su vez, estas células ayudan al sistema inmunológico, así como rejuvenecen los órganos, incluyendo la reconstrucción muscular. El programa de yoga que seguí se basa en la respiración y el movimiento. Me mantengo alerta de los patrones de sueño para obtener la salud máxima.

Mi profesor de yoga combina Ayurveda (dieta) y asanas (posiciones corporales) para llevar una vida saludable. El creó un yoga llamado kundalini tantra yoga que se centra en el movimiento (tantra yoga original) y la respiración (kundalini+prananyama). Sus rutinas se centran especialmente en el coxis y las caderas (región pélvica) y los hombros, para construir glóbulos rojos. De hecho, el utiliza un movimiento circular de los hombros y movimientos pélvicos circulares en muchas posiciones. Sólo después de estudiar sobre la médula ósea fui consciente de la ciencia de su yoga. Nos está diciendo constantemente que "la vida está en el coxis".

Mi maestro de yoga ha modificado la postura de yoga "perro boca abajo" enfatizando el movimiento para evitar la acumulación de sangre estancada en el cerebro combinada con más movimiento de la columna vertebral, y la acción del coxis. Su forma de posición de perro hacia abajo se practica con movimientos oscilantes. Esto ayuda a activar los hombros, la columna vertebral y el coxis al mismo tiempo.

Usé en la recuperación Equinácea en forma de tintura como un refuerzo inmune. Esta ha sido una herramienta poderosa en mi pasado como prevención en periodos de estrés. Sin embargo, parecía relevante en la recuperación dado el agotamiento de mi sistema inmunológico. Empecé en mayo, y terminaré en agosto (solo dos meses).

Los alimentos ricos en vitamina C a diario fueron especialmente importantes para mí. Comí una naranja por la mañana (espera de 20 minutos para digerir y transformarme en alcalina), bebí jugo de limón caliente al despertar, y antes del entrenamiento de yoga 1-2 kiwis. También tomé un suplemento de vitamina C durante el pico del virus durante 2 meses después del virus. Mi profesor de yoga me recomendó té de hierba de limón o papaya. No pude obtener estos artículos. Los tomates junto con los pimientos verdes pronto estarán en temporada. ¡Estos alimentos de forma natural fortalecerán mi sistema inmunológico, ya que se llenan del rico sol de la temporada de crecimiento del fresco verano de mi jardín!

Me acuesto lo suficientemente temprano como para dormir a las 10 de la noche. Si estoy cansada, me meto en la cama antes para compensar el tiempo de relajación, 1,5 horas antes. Si no estoy fatigada mentalmente, puedo deslizarme en el sueño fácilmente dentro de los 30-45 minutos siguientes. Me levanto temprano y me ocupo de mi jardín, el horario de un granjero, en armonía con el ritmo natural del sol. De hecho, me despierto antes del amanecer para obtener una energía óptima, y capitalizo la energía del sol que me impulsa hacia el día. Prefiero esta táctica a correr detrás del sol, levantándome tarde.

Masa muscular: La fiebre fue muy baja, pero los músculos me dolieron más que en pasadas ocasiones con una fiebre normal y escalofríos. Nunca tuve escalofríos o sudores por la noche. Estaba deshidratada por todo el proceso del virus. Mi masa corporal bajó 9 kilos (20 libras) en 3 semanas. A pesar de que comí carbohidratos y apenas realicé ejercicio. Estoy asombrada por la pérdida de grasa y músculo. Apenas podía caminar, y sentía que con la pérdida de los músculos de las piernas tenía que volver a aprender a caminar. En mis primeros días al ir de compras, recuerdo tener problemas para dar un paseo a solo 2 manzanas de distancia de la tienda de comestibles. Subir los 3 tramos de escaleras con las bolsas de la compra era arduo. Temía salir a buscar cualquier cosa, pero me había quedado sin alimentos frescos. Tardaba tanto en vestirme. No podía estar de pie más de 5 minutos.

También era una agonía en mis pies cocinar. Tenía que sentarme varias veces durante estas tareas ordinarias. Por no hablar de mi cerebro a cámara lenta. Tenía que preparar mi bolso, guantes, máscara, abrigo, zapatos y carrito de compras. Al regresar, tenía que quitarme la ropa y los zapatos en el hall de entrada, descargar el carro de la compra, limpiar todos los artículos y luego desinfectar el carro de la compra y los zapatos.

Nota: Por responsabilidad social, me había puesto en cuarentena 2 semanas después de que la fiebre disminuyese. Un amigo de Madrid amablemente vino a mi rescate con bolsas de comestibles, cuando me quedé sin frutas y verduras frescas después de 10 días. (Nuestro encierro estaba programado para 10 días, así que sólo compré suficiente para ese período). A toro pasado, habría cocinado comida y la habría congelado. En cuanto a las frutas frescas, las habría cortado y congelado o hecho batidos para congelar en bolsas de cierre hermético.

Parecía vital para mi cuerpo tener estos alimentos para alimentar mis músculos. Ver la nevera vacía no era una experiencia agradable. Normalmente me he defendido por mí misma, pero tuve que admitir que no tenía ni tiempo ni comida fresca. Más tarde me enteré de la red local de tiendas y vendedores que entregaban la compra a domicilio. Las grandes tiendas de comestibles tenían envío a domicilio, pero no tenían disponible el servicio de compra online. Fue complicado. Yo era nueva en la ciudad y no podía salir a preguntar a los vecinos.

Me sorprendió la pérdida de masa corporal en tan poco tiempo y la importancia del ejercicio para el sistema inmunológico. Leí algunos estudios sobre el tema y encontré lo siguiente:

- "Durante una infección, el cuerpo se vuelve catabólico (lo opuesto a anabólico) y descompone la proteína muscular. El grado de catabolismo muscular y pérdida de proteínas está relacionado con la altura y duración de la fiebre causada por la infección."
- "Los aminoácidos que se liberan en el músculo son eliminados por el hígado y utilizados como una fuente de energía de emergencia (producción de glucosa a través de la gluconeogénesis) y como bloques de construcción para las proteínas de fase aguda, que el cuerpo emplea para combatir la infección."
- "Los músculos tienen muchas buenas razones para te duelan cuando tienes una infección. El músculo esquelético es la principal fuente de proteína catabolizada, pero el músculo cardíaco también contribuye."
- "Los estudios han demostrado una disminución del 25 por ciento en la fuerza muscular isométrica después de una enfermedad febril simple como la gripe. Reponer la masa muscular perdida durante una enfermedad febril de tres días puede tardar hasta dos semanas."
- "De acuerdo con el ajuste del protocolo de ejercicio, puede causar micro traumas temporales de diferentes grados en los músculos esqueléticos [5, 6]. Estos micro traumas del músculo esquelético inducen el proceso de regeneración tisular. En este proceso, las células inmunitarias como neutrófilos y macrófagos se activan para trabajar en la recuperación de la homeostasis tisular, produciendo mediadores pro y antiinflamatorios."
- "En las últimas dos décadas, una variedad de estudios ha demostrado que el ejercicio induce un cambio fisiológico en el sistema inmunológico considerable. El ejercicio agudo y crónico altera el número y la función de las células circulantes

del sistema inmunitario innato (por ejemplo, neutrófilos, monocitos y células asesinas naturales (NK)."

- "Existe una relación directa entre el ejercicio y el sistema inmunitario. El ejercicio puede modular la respuesta del sistema inmunitario de forma aguda y crónica. Sin embargo, el ejercicio físico también induce a la liberación en la circulación sanguínea de mioquinas. La función fisiológica de las mioquinas producidas por el músculo esquelético es la de proteger y mejorar la funcionalidad de muchos órganos. Además, hay evidencia convincente de que los factores secretados por el músculo esquelético actúan como mediadores en la señalización endocrina y están involucrados en los efectos beneficiosos del ejercicio en casi todos los tipos de células y órganos."
- "Respuesta celular inmediatamente después del ejercicio. Observado un aumento significativo en la suma total de leucocitos, neutrófilos, monocitos y linfocitos inmediatamente después de los tres tipos de ejercicio. El ejercicio prolongado indujo a un mayor aumento en el recuento total de leucocitos circulantes, neutrófilos y monocitos, pero el pico del ejercicio aeróbico indujo a un aumento similar en el recuento de linfocitos; el ejercicio de resistencia provocó respuestas menores en todos los subconjuntos celulares."
- "Como un potente extensor de la articulación de la cadera, el Glúteo Máximus, que es adecuado para los poderosos movimientos de las extremidades inferiores como subir un escalón, escalar o correr, no se utiliza en gran medida durante la marcha normal. El Glúteo Máximus junto con los isquiotibiales trabajan juntos para extender el tronco desde una posición flexionada tirando de la pelvis hacia atrás, por ejemplo, de pie desde una posición inclinada hacia adelante. También proporcionan control excéntrico al doblar hacia delante. Las fibras superiores del Glúteo Máximo pueden extender la rodilla por su fijación al tracto Iliotibial."
- "El Glúteo Maximus tiene varios roles de estabilidad: mantener

el equilibrio de la pelvis en las cabezas femorales manteniendo así la postura erguida, su unión a través del tracto iliotibial apoya la rodilla lateral, y la rotación lateral del fémur cuando se está de pie ayuda a elevar el arco longitudinal medial del pie."

Recuperación: La producción de masa muscular para recuperar su pérdida tras su deterioro (un efecto secundario del virus) fue esencial. Después del 2 de mayo, cuando el encierro permitía el ejercicio al aire libre, las excursiones fueron parte de mi rutina diaria por la mañana temprano, principalmente con mi nueva bicicleta. ¡El aire fresco era celestial! No podía aguantar un paseo andando para hacer ejercicio cardiovascular. Eran demasiado difíciles las largas distancias y no sentía que mis pulmones o músculos se beneficiaran de paseos cortos, ni mi mente. El único inconveniente del paseo en bicicleta fue el elevado peso de la bicicleta en mi hombro en los 3 tramos de escaleras. Esto me llevó un poco de práctica y cada día me sentía más fuerte. Usé esta prueba de fuerza como un indicador de mi progreso para construir masa muscular.

Los entrenamientos de yoga para cardio fue lo primero que hice después del paseo en bicicleta o la excursión de ir de compras. Me preparé, especialmente con la carrera de obstáculos en la escalera para levantar la bicicleta o el carrito de la compra lleno de comestibles (kilos de frutas y verduras). Después del entrenamiento cardiovascular, hice posiciones de yoga para tonificar los músculos y ligamentos. Luego terminé con el pranayama "respiración de fuego" y yoga específico para el rejuvenecimiento de órganos (riñón, hígado, bazo) y la vía digestiva. Seguí el programa del mi maestro de yoga en Kundalini Tantra yoga. Al principio, sólo podía hacer 30 minutos divididos a partes iguales entre cardio (12 min) y respiración de fuego (8 min), tonificación (7 min). Nota: Era importante hacer la tonificación de cardio y muscular antes de la respiración de pranayama porque la liberación de las toxinas (pranayama) es mejor después de que la sangre se caliente / fluya y las articulaciones se lubriquen.

Tras 6 semanas de ejercicio, a mediados de julio, pude caminar 10 kilómetros (6 millas) sin fatigarme. Sentí que mis piernas se habían recuperado y los pulmones también. A menudo doy un paseo por la tarde después del almuerzo, y continúo el paseo en bicicleta a la granja eco temprano por la mañana disfrutando del aire fresco. Pesaba cerca de 59 kilos (132 libras) al principio y ahora 51 (113 libras) a mediados de julio. ¡De hecho me siento más joven y vibrante con mi nueva masa corporal! Mi yoga ha mejorado tremendamente con un cuerpo más ligero, especialmente la pérdida de la masa muscular más grande, Glúteo Maximus.

Mente:

La actitud durante este calvario fue clave para el resultado de tomar decisiones y controlar cómo abordar las situaciones que iban surgiendo. Mi cuerpo estaba sufriendo y sometido a tensión luchando con síntomas muy cambiantes. Un virus "novedoso" significa que se apodera de mi ser con un curso desconocido tanto para mi mente como para mi cuerpo. Tuve años de práctica con resfriados, tos, gripe, malestar estomacal, dolor muscular y muchas otras condiciones con las que he tenido que lidiar en el pasado. Sin embargo, este virus corrió una secuencia que era totalmente extraña para mí. No podía predecir cómo prepararme para cada nueva fase. De hecho, era imposible confrontarlo con experiencias pasadas y sin un patrón. Definitivamente el factor miedo forma parte del Covid-19 que está presente en algunos momentos más que en otros. Incluso si vas al hospital, ¿cómo pueden ayudarte? Aparte de los cuidados de emergencia, sin antibióticos ni cura, tuve que enfrentarme a cada fase simplemente a medida que iba golpeando a mi cuerpo. Sin embargo, estoy convencida de que mi mentalidad desde el principio fue una bendición gracias a mi maestro de yoga y a mis amigos. Creo que los tres elementos más importantes de mi mentalidad fueron 1) Risas, 2) Inspiración y 3) Mindfulness.

Risa

A principios de la semana ya había perdido algún contrato debido a Covid-19 y antes de que tuviera mi primer síntoma, la fiebre. Había entrado en una espiral descendente de negatividad y estragos emocionales de preocupación. Eso duró 2 días antes de salirme de ese agujero y de que empezara a pensar diferente. Ahora tenía más tiempo y el tiempo estaba precioso. Esto fue antes del encierro. Compré una bicicleta y empecé a montar por el campo. Tuve más tiempo para dedicarme al yoga y poner mi casa en orden después de un arduo horario invernal de desplazamientos a Madrid. Me sentía bastante positiva entrando en el confinamiento. Además, acababa de ver un breve videoclip de mi profesor de yoga con una sonrisa y riendo al hablar del Covid-19. Estaba exponiendo que nuestros cuerpos son como un contenedor para procesar lo negativo, así que había que dejar que siguiese su curso. Lo veía como un proceso de aprendizaje de cuánto se puede procesar negativo sin que a uno le afecte. También comentó: "Sé inteligente". Se reía, de hecho, para ayudarnos a tener menos miedo. Funcionó conmigo.

En los primeros días de fiebre y dolor de piernas estaba manteniendo una actitud jovial con el fin de procesar lo negativo y dejar que fluyera a través de mí. De hecho, era doloroso e incómodo, pero la cara y la sonrisa de mi profesor de yoga se me habían quedado grabadas. En realidad, no se lo dije a mucha gente. No quería ser victimista. Mi casero dijo en broma que su hermana "probablemente lo tenía, y todos terminaríamos por cogerlo ". Él también le quitaba importancia. Resultó que tanto su hermana como su hija de dos años lo tenían, pero lo pasaron de forma suave. En fin, tanto mi profesor de yoga como mi casero fueron desde el principio los dos faros que me iluminaron al respecto. Los imité y comencé a concentrarme en la risa.

Me había acordado de un médico oncólogo que recomendaba videos o libros divertidos para ayudar al cerebro a mantenerse animado durante la quimioterapia y todo el proceso de la enfermedad. Cómo el cerebro reacciona a las situaciones es realmente importante para crear así una cadena de reacciones químicas en el cuerpo. La risa produce endorfinas que estimulan el sistema inmunitario o al menos no lo agotan.

Empecé a pedir a mis amigos que me enviaran sólo chistes de las redes sociales y que dejasen fuera las noticias políticas o deprimentes del virus. Hubo un montón de controversias políticas circulando por internet enredando a la gente en el debate. Quería mantener alejado de mi cerebro ese tipo de carga. La mayoría de la gente fue atenta y dejó de enviar mensajes de este tipo. Tuve algunos amigos que realmente estaban atentos a enviarme al menos una broma al día, o más. Yo agradecía estos mensajes. Los reenviaba a otros y todos nos reíamos. Incluso los traduje para que otros los disfrutaran. Los españoles son muy inteligentes e ingeniosos, con Don Quijote como referente. Los vídeos e imágenes caseros eran graciosísimos. ¡Estaba sola en mi cuarentena, pero riéndome en voz alta! Obtenía una buena dosis de risas diaria, unas cuantas veces al día. Siento que esta actitud fue esencial a la hora de mantener mi cuerpo reaccionando de manera favorable a cada fase.

Inspiración

La inspiración se presenta de diferentes maneras. En la formación de liderazgo se llama motivación. En la curación se llama afirmaciones. En los deportes se llama "hacer otra vuelta" y luego tirar el tiro libre (cuando estás cansado). He estado expuesta a todos estos tipos de inspiración y más. En yoga es un poco diferente. Se llama Bhakti yoga. Te ofreces a ti mismo y esto inspira a otros a hacer lo mismo. Se modela desde la luna. Como la luna sólo refleja la luz del sol, ofreciendo un recipiente para una luz en la oscuridad. Un faro tiene la misma función. Este tipo de inspiración es el primer paso hacia los demás y luego crea un efecto domino. Finalmente vuelve como amor del universo y tal vez de otros.

Empecé a enviar mensajes de texto inspiradores por la mañana y por la noche en las redes sociales. Me iba a la cama temprano y me levantaba también temprano con los pájaros, así que empecé con esta imagen. Busqué pájaros hermosos como símbolo de la primavera. Enviaba un mensaje de "Good morning, Buenos Días". Por la noche buscaba relajantes imágenes de puestas de sol con "Good night, Buenos Días". También era una manera de estar pendiente de todos los que me importaban. Creé mi "tribu" de forma individual y no como grupo de WhatsApp. Quería respetar la privacidad de las personas. ¡Llevó un poco de tecleo de los dedos, pero mereció la pena!

Durante la pandemia, la gente parecía estar aburrida, inquieta y preocupada por aumentar de peso. Les enviaba bailes divertidos, recetas o música para animarlos a ser positivos. La gente respondía y eliminábamos nuestras preocupaciones chateando. Realmente agradecía todos esos mensajes y el esfuerzo que la gente realizó para mantenerme animada. También se aseguraron de que estuviera bien. Estoy segura de que estaban preocupados. Parecía haber un sinfín de hermosos pájaros con flores de primavera para enviar diariamente. ¡Incluso grabé el canto de los pájaros de mi ventana! Cambié a flores de loto, mariposas, caballos y otras imágenes de la naturaleza. Me parecía que la música clásica como Handel era muy inspiradora. Con todo, estaba muy agradecida por "mi tribu" y por la inspiración mutua que compartíamos. Es el final de julio y todavía estoy enviando "Buenos días" casi todos los días.

Mindfulness

Se dice que el mindfulness (atención plena) es un concepto original del budismo. Buda, habiendo sido un yogui luchando por la mejor manera de llegar al final del sufrimiento, descubrió "el camino medio". El camino medio significa no ser extremo y se centra en el PRESENTE, ni en el pasado ni en el futuro. El concepto de mindfulness de estar en el "ahora" es una reacción a la ansiedad que enfrentamos en un estilo de vida moderno que requiere varias habilidades para mitigar el rápido ritmo diario, especialmente en entornos urbanos.

En el pasado, una persona hiperactiva se consideraba anormal. ¡Hoy en día este comportamiento "normal" se llama "multitarea" y es una destreza que se recompensa! El hiper estilo de vida está sacado de quicio por un mercado global que supera los límites de nuestra capacidad humana para mantenerse al día con las últimas tendencias o productividad. Nosotros mismos, incluida yo misma, programamos y llenamos nuestros horarios con poco descanso o espacio para siquiera concentrarnos en la presente tarea antes de pasar al siguiente objetivo (ya sea mental o físicamente).

En el escenario Covid-19, me vi obligada a utilizar mindfulness debido a mi falta de energía y limitada mi actividad cerebral. Me fue muy útil recordar cómo ralentizar la mente. Había aprendido esta habilidad en la meditación. Mi maestro de yoga, me enseñó a no preocuparme por la mente divagando, sino a dejarla ir. Él me recomendó el concepto de pantalla dividida. En otras palabras, no trates de usar la mente para calmar la mente (casi imposible). Él se centraba en el corazón. Escuchas tu corazón y te centras en su conexión con el universo. A medida que el enfoque sobre corazón aumenta, la mente disminuye. Sólo tenía que mantener mi mente centrada para evitar distracciones.

Me di cuenta de que la mente siempre está reaccionando a los estímulos externos o señales visuales que la distraen. Tuve que resistir a mi mente que miraba hacia un rincón de la casa con suciedad y quería limpiarla. Estaba atraída por sus impulsos a poner una lavadora después de limpiar el baño. Era el momento de bajar la marcha. Tuve que establecer horarios para mantenerme saludable. Hoy estoy lavando la ropa, lo que significa simplemente darle al interruptor y esperar a descargar y colgarla para secar. Mañana voy a fregar el suelo o desempolvarlos. Al día siguiente voy a hacer el baño (solamente lo esencial) y sin una limpieza en profundad. Mantuve mi mente a raya para no acumular tareas en un sólo día. Reparto las tareas domésticas.

La cocina también supuso un punto de inflexión en el mindfulness. Tuve que crear un par de recetas sencillas para el desayuno y el almuerzo. Después del almuerzo no tenía más energía. Opté por un plato de frutas, pelando un plátano y cortando otra pieza de fruta. Esto me ahorró tiempo de lavado los platos después de la cena. El desayuno era lento y sin prisas. Dejé el café y eso me ayudó a estar menos ansiosa. Teniendo en cuenta que no tenía nada que hacer y a ningún lugar donde ir, el café estaba sobrevalorado. El cortar verduras me exigió mucha concentración para evitar cortarme los dedos. Así que lo hice lenta y uniformemente. No estaba segura de lo bien que mi sistema podría manejar un corte o infección. También las ollas y sartenes se mantuvieron bajo mínimos. Usé un plato, un tazón, una cuchara, un tenedor y dos cuchillos. No dejé ningún plato sucio por la noche y menos vajilla que era fácil de lavar.

Me sentía como si estuviera viviendo en una larga meditación. La casa estaba en silencio, la comunidad estaba en silencio, las calles estaban en silencio. Sin embargo, eso no garantizaba que la mente se callara. Tenía que estar alerta y vigilar los desvíos. A veces ponía música clásica suave para inspirarme. Canté mantras de forma jovial para mantener mi mente distraída para conectar con el universo. Tuve suerte de haber desarrollado ya algunas habilidades para la meditación. Sin embargo, el virus me puso a prueba. Tuve que aplicar todo mi conocimiento desde diferentes planos para superar una crisis mental, especialmente aguantando el virus sola en aislamiento.

References

"Coronaviruses are able to infect bone marrow cells, resulting in abnormal hematopoiesis. Hematopoiesis: The production of all types of blood cells including formation, development, and differentiation of blood cells. Hematopoiesis is the production of all of the cellular components of blood and blood plasma. It occurs within the hematopoietic system, which includes organs and tissues such as the bone marrow, liver, and spleen. Simply, hematopoiesis is the process through which the body manufactures blood cells. In adults, hematopoiesis of red blood cells and platelets occurs primarily in the bone marrow." (Pascutti: 2016).

- Pascutti, M. F., Erkelens, M. N., & Nolte, M. A. (2016). Impact of Viral Infections on Hematopoiesis: From Beneficial to Detrimental Effects on Bone Marrow Output. *Frontiers in immunology*, 7, 364. https://doi.org/10.3389/fimmu.2016.00364

"A low white blood cell count usually is caused by: Viral infections that temporarily disrupt the work of bone marrow." (Mayo Clinic: Retrieved, July 2020).

- https://www.mayoclinic.org/symptoms/low-white-blood-cell-count/basics/causes/sym-20050615

"Bone marrow is the tissue comprising the centre of large bones. Damaged pulmonary capillary beds cause the process of megakaryocyte rupture and platelet release to be blocked, which affects the release of platelets into the pulmonary circulation and indirectly leads to reduced platelet synthesis in the systemic circulation." (Zucher-Franklin & Philipp: 2000).

- Zucker-Franklin, D., & Philipp, C. S. (2000). Platelet production in the pulmonary capillary bed: new ultrastructural evidence for an old concept. *The American journal of pathology*, 157(1), 69–74. https://doi.org/10.1016/S0002-9440(10)64518-X

"The bone marrow is where new blood cells are produced. Bone marrow contains two types of stem cells: hemopoietic (which can produce blood cells) and stromal (which can produce fat, cartilage and bone). There are two types of bone marrow: red marrow (also known as myeloid tissue) and yellow marrow. Red blood cells, platelets and most white blood cells arise in red marrow; some white blood cells develop in yellow marrow. The colour of yellow marrow is due to the much higher number of fat cells." (Science Daily: Retrieved, July 2020)

- https://www.sciencedaily.com/terms/bone_marrow.htm

"In cases of severe blood loss, the body can convert yellow marrow back to red marrow in order to increase blood cell production. Lack of red blood cells causes the body to draw from yellow marrow to convert back to red marrow to produce red blood cells (oxygen carriers). Yellow marrow is designed to produce fat and tissue after the age of five. Fat and muscle mass reduction result from inactivity (bed ridden-muscle mass loss) and lack of production from yellow marrow (fat cells) in order to help red blood marrow, produce healthy red cells."

- https://www.britannica.com/science/bone-marrow
- https://www.newworldencyclopedia.org/entry/Bone_marrow
- https://www.msdmanuals.com/home/blood-disorders/biology-of-blood/components-of-blood

"Red blood cells, white blood cells, and platelets are all produced in the red bone marrow. As we age, the distribution of red and yellow bone marrow changes. Bone marrow's highest production in adults is located in the shoulder, pelvic and spine areas of the human body bone structure."

"A low white blood cell count usually means your body isn't making enough white blood cells. It can increase your risk of all sorts of infections. Some groups, such as people of Afro-Caribbean and Middle Eastern descent, often have a low white blood cell count but this is normal and doesn't increase their risk of infections."

"Neutrophils are the first defense against invading microorganisms. Increased susceptibility to common pathogens has usually been attributed to extremely low counts (below 0.5×109/l) (13) and individuals with "low normal" counts or ethnic neutropenia have not been reported to be at increased risk as long as counts are not further decreased. However, the probability to contract tuberculosis from patients with open pulmonary disease was inversely correlated with baseline neutrophil counts in a recent study."

"Neutrophil counts in blood are determined by the differentiation and proliferation of precursor cells in the bone marrow, release of mature neutrophils into the blood, margination in organs like the lung and spleen, and transmigration through the endothelial lining followed by neutrophil apoptosis and uptake by phagocytes. One example is benign ethnic neutropenia, which is found in about 5% of African Americans. Reduced and elevated neutrophil counts, even within the normal range, are associated with excess all-cause mortality."

- https://microbenotes.com/bone-marrow-types-structure-and-functions/
- https://open.oregonstate.education/aandp/chapter/6-1-the-functions-of-the-skeletal-system/
- https://www.leukaemia.org.au/blood-cancer-information/types-of-blood-cancer/understanding-your-blood/bone-marrow-and-blood-formation/
- https://www.nhs.uk/conditions/low-white-blood-cell-count/
- https://www.ncbi.nlm.nih.gov/pmc/articles/PMC2745132/
- von Vietinghoff, S., & Ley, K. (2008). Homeostatic regulation of blood neutrophil counts. *Journal of immunology (Baltimore, Md.: 1950)*, *181*(8), 5183–5188. https://doi.org/10.4049/jimmunol.181.8.5183

"Our bodies don't make vitamin C, but we need it for immune function, bone structure, iron absorption, and healthy skin. We get vitamin C from our diet, usually in citrus fruits, strawberries, green vegetables, and tomatoes." (Harvard: January 17, 2020).

- https://www.health.harvard.edu/cold-and-flu/can-vitamin-c-prevent-a-cold

"Sleep plays a major role in repair work on the human body. There's a substantial body of evidence that stress weakens the immune system and makes us vulnerable to infection and disease. a relationship between sleep and a healthy immune system, and the damage that a lack of sleep can have. While more sleep won't necessarily prevent you from getting sick, skimping on it could adversely affect your immune system, The immune system kicks into action during that time."

- https://www.sleepfoundation.org/articles/how-sleep-affects-your-immunity
- https://www.psychologytoday.com/us/blog/sleep-newzzz/201208/lack-sleep-dangerous-stress-healthy-immune-function

"During an infection, the body becomes catabolic (the opposite of anabolic) and breaks down muscle protein. The degree of muscle catabolism and protein loss is related to the height and duration of the fever caused by the infection. The amino acids that are liberated from muscle are scavenged by the liver and used as an emergency energy source (glucose production via gluconeogenesis) and as the building blocks for acute phase proteins, which the body employs to fight infection. Your muscles have many good reasons to ache when you have an infection. Skeletal muscle is the main source of catabolized protein, but heart muscle contributes as well."

"Studies have shown a 25 percent decrease in isometric muscle strength after a simple febrile illness such as the flu. Replenishing muscle mass lost during a three-day febrile illness may take up to two weeks."

"As a powerful extensor of the hip joint, the gluteus maximus suited to powerful lower limb movements such as stepping onto a step, climbing or running but is not used greatly during normal walking. Gluteus maximus and the hamstrings work together to extend the trunk from a flexed position by pulling the pelvis backwards, for example standing up from a bent forward position. Eccentric control is also provided when bending forward. Superior fibres of the gluteus maximus can extend the knee through its attachment to the Iliotibial tract."

"Gluteus maximus has several stability roles: balancing the pelvis on femoral heads thus maintaining upright posture, the attachment through the iliotibial tract supports the lateral knee, and lateral rotation of femur when standing assists raising the medial longitudinal arch of the foot."

- https://www.ncbi.nlm.nih.gov/books/NBK224630/
- Jain, S., Gautam, V., & Naseem, S. (2011). Acute-phase proteins: As diagnostic tool. *Journal of pharmacy & bioallied sciences*, *3*(1), 118–127. https://doi.org/10.4103/0975-7406.76489
- Cruzat, V., Macedo Rogero, M., Noel Keane, K., Curi, R., & Newsholme, P. (2018). Glutamine: Metabolism and Immune Function, Supplementation and Clinical Translation. *Nutrients*, *10*(11), 1564. https://doi.org/10.3390/nu10111564
- https://www.active.com/health/articles/scare-tactics-to-prevent-you-from-exercising-while-sick
- https://www.physio-pedia.com/Gluteus_Maximus
- Kinesiology of the Hip: A Focus on Muscular Actions. Donald A. Neumann. Journal of Orthopaedic & Sports Physical Therapy 2010 40:2, 82-94. https://www.jospt.org/doi/10.2519/jospt.2010.3025

"Turmeric, a spice that has long been recognized for its medicinal properties, has received interest from both the medical/scientific world and from culinary enthusiasts, as it is the major source of the polyphenol curcumin. It aids in the management of oxidative and inflammatory conditions, metabolic syndrome, arthritis, anxiety, and hyperlipidemia."

"It may also help in the management of exercise-induced inflammation and muscle soreness, thus enhancing recovery and performance in active people. In addition, a relatively low dose of the complex can provide health benefits for people that do not have diagnosed health conditions. Most of these benefits can be attributed to its antioxidant and anti-inflammatory effects."

"Ingesting curcumin by itself does not lead to the associated health benefits due to its poor bioavailability, which appears to be primarily due to poor absorption, rapid metabolism, and rapid elimination. There are several components that can increase bioavailability. For example, piperine is the major active component of black pepper and, when combined in a complex with curcumin, has been shown to increase bioavailability by 2000%."

"Curcumin, a polyphenol, has been shown to target multiple signaling molecules while also demonstrating activity at the cellular level, which has helped to support its multiple health benefits. It has been shown to benefit inflammatory conditions, metabolic syndrome, pain], and to help in the management of inflammatory and degenerative eye conditions. In addition, it has been shown to benefit the kidneys."

- https://www.ncbi.nlm.nih.gov/pmc/articles/PMC5664031/
- Hewlings, S. J., & Kalman, D. S. (2017). Curcumin: A Review of Its' Effects on Human Health. *Foods (Basel, Switzerland)*, 6(10), 92. https://doi.org/10.3390/foods6100092

"There are several plausible mechanisms that suggest favorable effect of curcumin on liver function. Curcumin might ameliorate hepatic steatosis and block fatty liver disease progression through inhibiting fatty acids synthesis and biosynthesis of unsaturated fatty acids such as stearic acid, oleic acid and linoleic acid.33 It can improve mitochondrial activity, facilitate β-oxidation and decrease lipogenesis.34 In addition, reports have indicated that oxidative stress and immune system disorder plays important roles in contribute to liver dysfunction such as NAFLD.35 In this case, curcumin can improve oxidative stress and prevent NAFLD by decrease production of reactive oxygen species, the hepatic protein expression of oxidative stress, pro-inflammatory cytokines, and chemokines such as interferon (IFN) γ, interleukin-1β and IFNγ-inducible protein 10.36, 37." Curcumin, which constitutes 2–5% of turmeric, is perhaps the most-studied component. Although some of the activities of turmeric can be mimicked by curcumin, other activities are curcumin-"

"Cell-based studies have demonstrated the potential of turmeric as an antimicrobial, insecticidal, larvicidal, antimutagenic, radioprotector, and anticancer agent. Turmeric has also been used to support liver function and to treat jaundice in both Ayurvedic and Chinese herbal medicine."

"Research during the past decade has identified numerous chemical entities from turmeric, and modern science has provided a logical basis for the safety and efficacy of turmeric against human diseases. Epidemiologic data indicate that some extremely common cancers in the Western world are much less prevalent in regions (Southeast Asia, e.g.) where turmeric is widely consumed in the diet. spice has been found well tolerated at gram doses in humans. Dietary turmeric contains over 300 different components."

- http://www.sciencedirect.com/science/article/pii/S2213422018301069
- Fariborz Mansour-Ghanaei, et al. (2019) Efficacy of curcumin/turmeric on liver enzymes in patients with non-alcoholic fatty liver disease: A systematic review of randomized

controlled trials, Integrative Medicine Research, Volume 8, Issue1, https://doi.org/10.1016/j.imr.2018.07.004

- https://onlinelibrary.wiley.com/doi/full/10.1002/mnfr.201100741?casa_token=rpAC9nnzVEYAAAAA%3AWF-NaDRmVRiWD_AKpGl-RgUosV03fiPjwkXVmn-wra_aXx8rZPRAyanQFMr5lc-Ur6HgiXKiYdBuwz40U
- Gupta, S.C., Sung, B., Kim, J.H., Prasad, S., Li, S. and Aggarwal, B.B. (2013), Multitargeting by turmeric, the golden spice: From kitchen to clinic. Mol. Nutr. Food Res., 57: 1510-1528. doi:10.1002/mnfr.201100741

"During an infection, the body becomes catabolic (the opposite of anabolic) and breaks down muscle protein. The degree of muscle catabolism and protein loss is related to the height and duration of the fever caused by the infection."

"The amino acids that are liberated from muscle are scavenged by the liver and used as an emergency energy source (glucose production via gluconeogenesis) and as the building blocks for acute phase proteins, which the body employs to fight infection."

"Your muscles have many good reasons to ache when you have an infection. Skeletal muscle is the main source of catabolized protein, but heart muscle contributes as well."

"According to the adjustment of the exercise protocol, it can cause temporary microtraumas of varying degrees in skeletal muscles. These skeletal muscle microtraumas induce the tissue regeneration process. In this process, immune cells such as neutrophils and macrophages are activated to work in the recovery of tissue homeostasis, producing pro- and anti-inflammatory mediators."

"Over the past two decades, a variety of studies has demonstrated that exercise induces considerable physiological change in the immune system. Acute and chronic exercise alters the number and function of circulating cells of the innate immune system (e.g., neutrophils, monocytes, and natural killer (NK) cells)."

"There is a straight relationship between exercise and the immune system. Exercise may modulate the immune system response acutely and chronically. Nevertheless, physical exercise also induces the release of myokines in the blood circulation. The physiological function of myokines produced by the skeletal muscle is to protect and improve the functionality of many organs. Furthermore, there is convincing evidence that factors secreted by the skeletal muscle act as endocrine signaling mediators and are involved in the beneficial effects of exercise on almost all cell types and organs."

"Cellular response immediately after exercise. We observed a significant increase in total leukocyte, neutrophil, monocyte and lymphocyte counts immediately following all three types of exercise. Prolonged exercise induced the greatest increase in total circulating leukocyte, neutrophil and monocyte counts, but peak aerobic exercise induced a similar increase in lymphocyte counts; lesser responses in all cell subsets were provoked by resistance exercise."

- https://www.hindawi.com/journals/jir/2018/9675216/
- Fortunato, et al. (2018) Strength Training Session Induces Important Changes on Physiological, Immunological, and Inflammatory Biomarkers. Journal of Immunology Research. Volume 2018 |Article ID 9675216. https://doi.org/10.1155/2018/9675216.
- https://www.scielo.br/pdf/spmj/v121n1/16127.pdf
- Effects of three different types of exercise on blood leukocyte count during and following exercise.

Ecological Dimensions of the *Ramayana*: A Conversation with Paula Richman. P. 31. The *Trumpeter,* ISSN: 0832-6193, Volume 25, Number 1 (2009).

- https://scholar.google.com/citations?user=s95_nVkAAAAJ&hl=en
- http://trumpeter.athabascau.ca/index.php/trumpet/article/view/1150

"People who eat chili peppers on a regular basis appear to lower their risk of dying from heart disease, a new study finds. Researchers analyzed the diets and health records of more than 22,000 people living in southern Italy and followed them for a median of just over eight years. People who ate chili peppers more than four times a week were about one-third less likely to die of heart disease than those who rarely or never ate the spicy-hot peppers. This protective benefit was evident regardless of whether people followed a Mediterranean-style diet (which is often recommended for heart health) or a less healthful diet. Chili peppers get their heat from a compound called capsaicin, which may help dampen inflammation and other harmful processes involved in the buildup of fatty plaque in arteries, according to the authors. Their study appeared Dec. 24, 2019, in the *Journal of the American College of Cardiology*." (Harvard University, March 2020).

- https://www.health.harvard.edu/heart-health/chili-peppers-the-spice-of-a-longer-life

"When you bite into a pepper, the capsaicin attaches to a receptor that communicates with other cells. That communication causes a nerve on your tongue to immediately tell your brain that it's hot. That same receptor is found in your digestive tract. When capsaicin enters your digestive tract and attaches to the receptor, it creates a chemical called anandamide. Anandamide has been shown to lead to less inflammation in the gut, which can be caused by conditions such as ulcerative colitis and Crohn's disease. The same reaction that calms down your gastrointestinal tract may also keep it tumor-free. It may be particularly effective for people that are at high risk of developing intestinal tumors — such as people with a family or personal history of tumors." (University of Pennsylvania 2019).

- https://www.pennmedicine.org/updates/blogs/health-and-wellness/2019/april/spicy-foods

Kundalini Tantra Yoga

"This is a technique and system of healing which comes from Mr. Arsana's personal mastery of Yoga and yearning to find the best method of healing the body. By combining flowing movements and specific breathing techniques it raises the energy within your body and activates your glands to regenerate. You heal from within and become more flexible, not only physically but your mental state of flow too." Developed and mastered by Mahatma Healer, Guru Ketut Arsana."

- https://www.omhamretreat.com/bali-yoga/

Colour psychology

"Seafoam green is one of the softest colors associated with the ocean. With notes of green and blue, but also with a small tint of grey.

"This color adds grey but is interestingly the color that has the most green within it. This means that the overall mood of the color is affected largely by the nature notes of green, but it does not overshadow the softness of the color, leaving it refreshingly bright green."

"The color seafoam green actually has a lot of positive associations and feelings attached to it. This color is mostly seen as connecting to the sea, and because of the softness and brightness of it, it is also often used when the room is needing a bit of cheering up, or when you need to feel a little more fresh and soft".

- What is seafoam's psychological qualities? (2020) https://www.colorpsychology.org/seafoam/

Turquoise:

"This is a color that recharges our spirits during times of mental stress and tiredness, alleviating feelings of loneliness. You only have to focus on the color turquoise, whether on a wall or clothing and you feel instant calm and gentle invigoration, ready to face the world again!"

"It is a great color to have around you, particularly in an emergency, as it helps with clear thinking and decision-making. It assists in the development of organizational and management skills."

"Turquoise encourages inner healing through its ability to enhance empathy and caring. It heightens our intuitive ability and opens the door to spiritual growth. It is the color of the evolved soul."

- *Turquoise means open communication and clarity of thought* (2018) https://www.empower-yourself-with-color-psychology.com/color-turquoise.html